high fit home

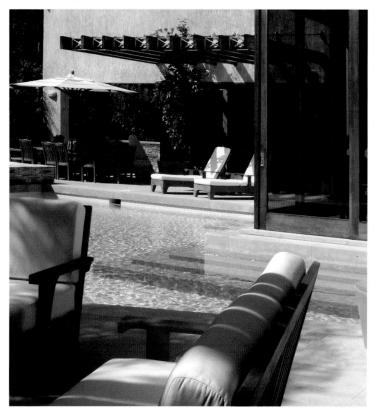

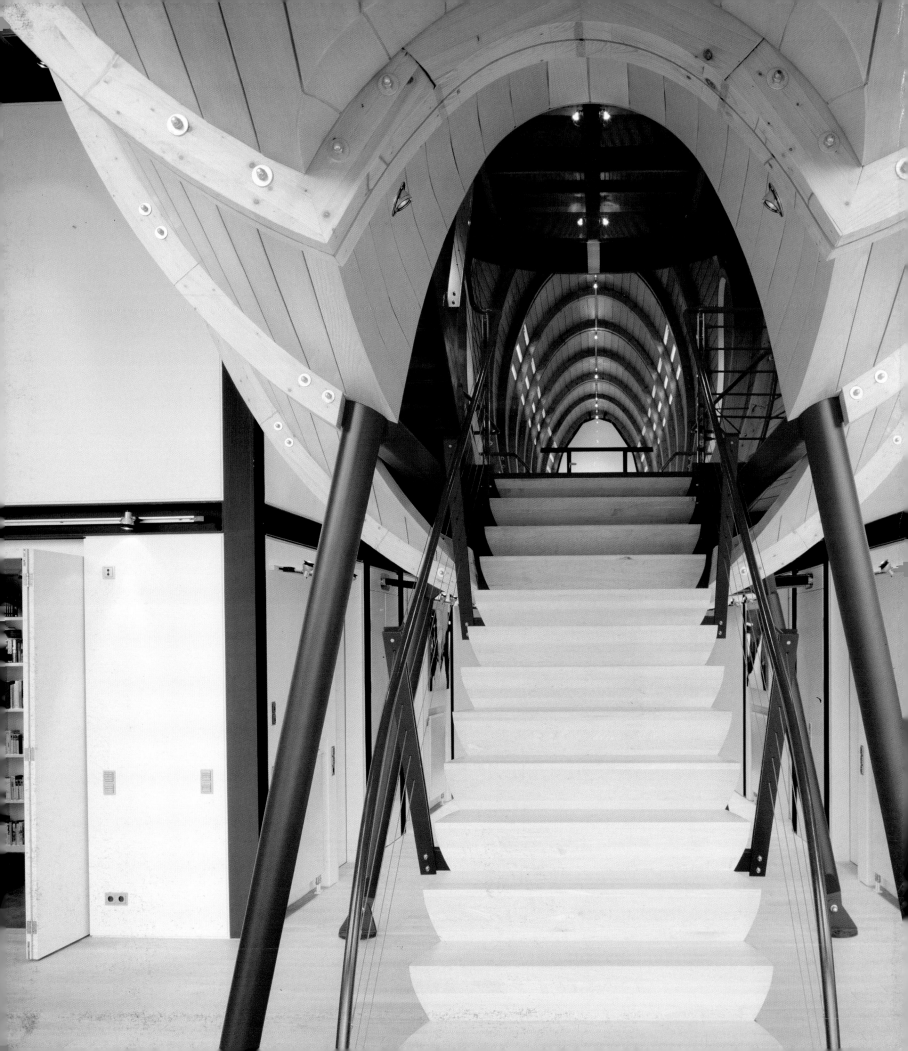

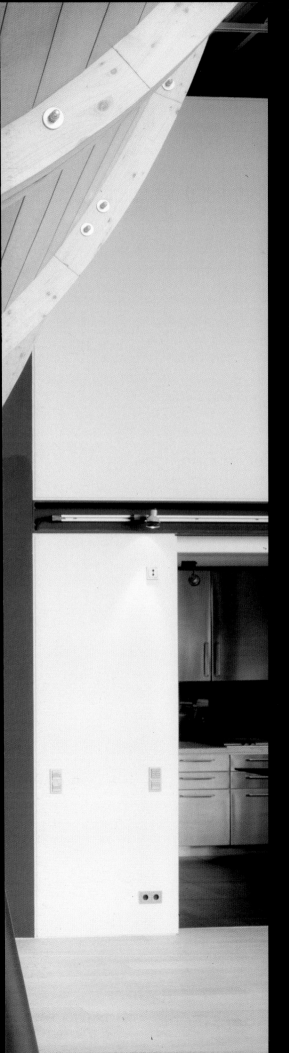

high fit home

DESIGNING YOUR HOME FOR HEALTH AND FITNESS

JOAN VOS MACDONALD

HARPER DESIGN

An Imprint of HarperCollins*Publishers*

HIGH FIT HOME: Designing Your Home for Health and Fitness
Copyright © 2005 by
GLITTERATI INCORPORATED
www.GlitteratiIncorporated.com

Text copyright © 2005 by Joan Vos MacDonald

First published in 2005 by:
Harper Design,
An Imprint of HarperCollins*Publishers*
10 East 53rd Street
New York, NY 10022
Tel: (212) 207-7000
Fax: (212) 207-7654
HarperDesign@harpercollins.com
www.harpercollins.com

Distributed throughout the world by:
HarperCollins International
10 East 53rd Street
New York, NY 10022
Fax: (212) 207-7654

HarperCollins books may be purchased for educational,
business, or sales promotional use. For information, please
write: Special Markets Department, HarperCollins
Publishers Inc., 10 East 53rd Street, New York, NY 10022.

Design: Susi Oberhelman

Library of Congress Cataloging-in-Publication Data

MacDonald, Joan Vos.
    High fit home: designing your home for health and
fitness / by Joan Vos MacDonald.
        p. cm.
    Includes index.
    ISBN 0-06-075161-4 (hardcover)
    1. Housing and health. 2. Architecture, Domestic—
Planning. 3. Architecture, Domestic—Health aspects.
4. Home gyms—Design and construction. 5. Physical
fitness centers—Design and construction. 6. Architecture,
Modern—20th century. 7. Architectural design. I. Title.

    RA770.M335 2004
    728'0246137—dc22   2004027750

FIRST EDITION

Printed and bound in China

1 2 3 4 5 6 7 / 11 10 09 08 07 06 05

FIRST PRINTING, 2005

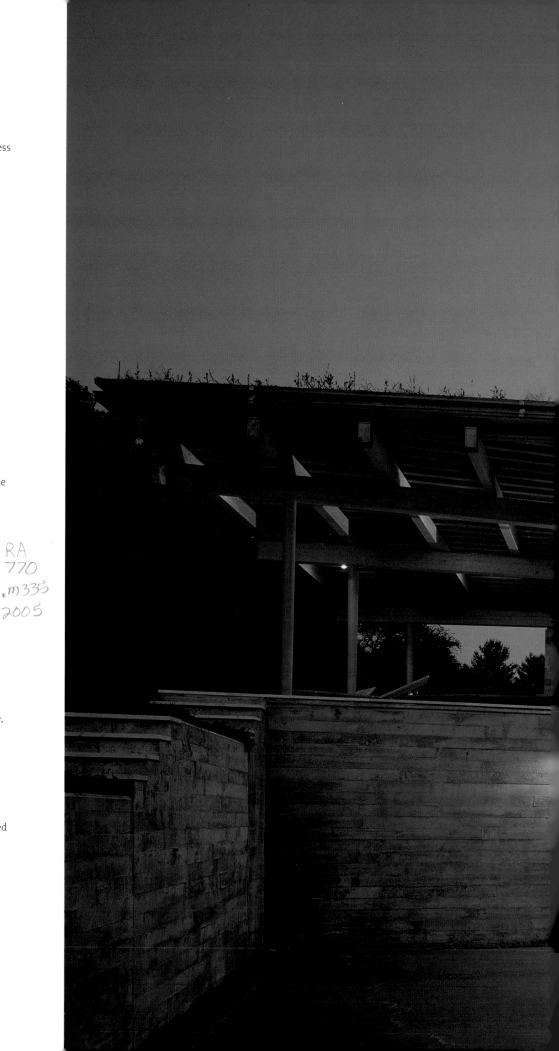

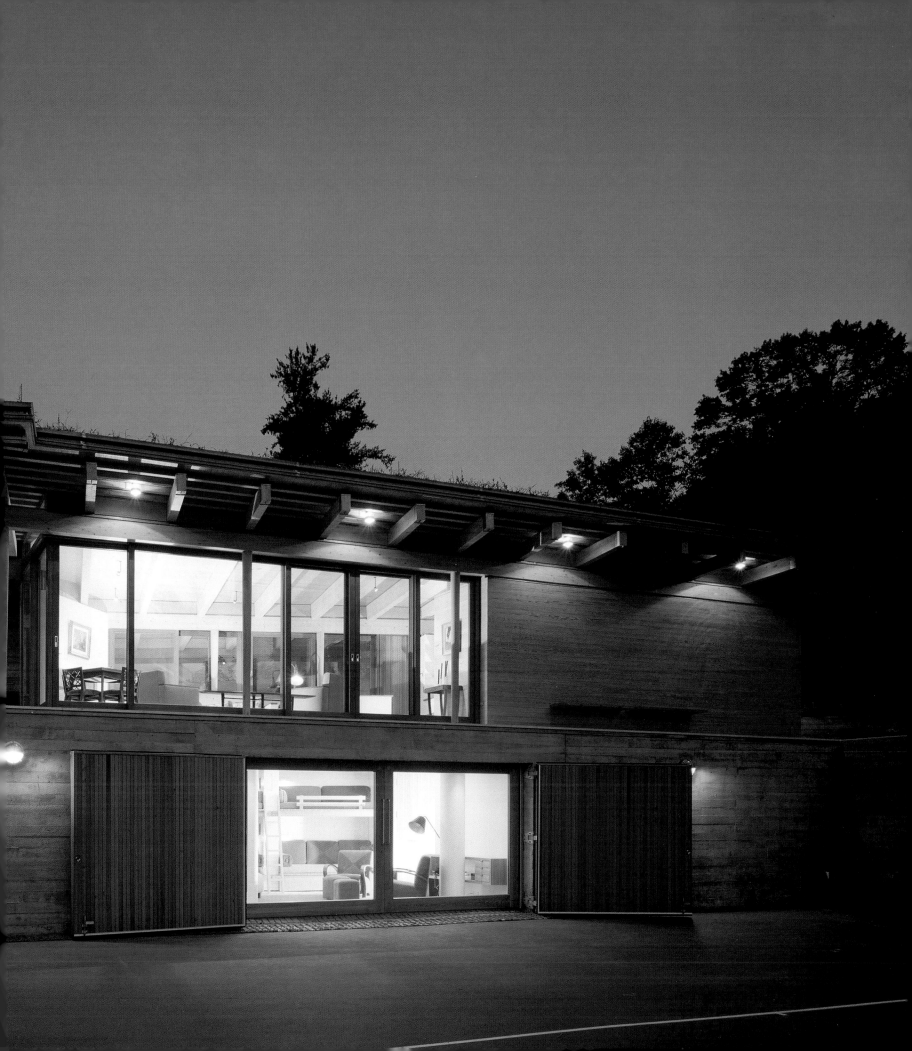

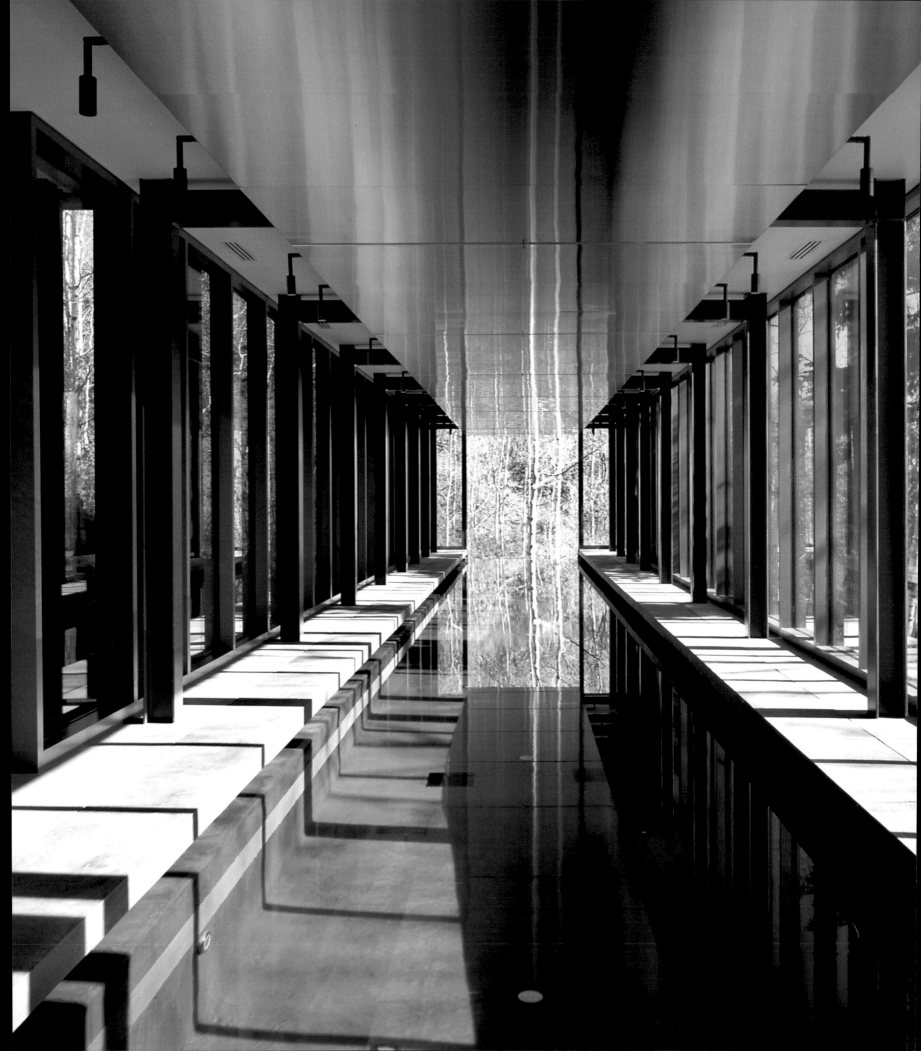

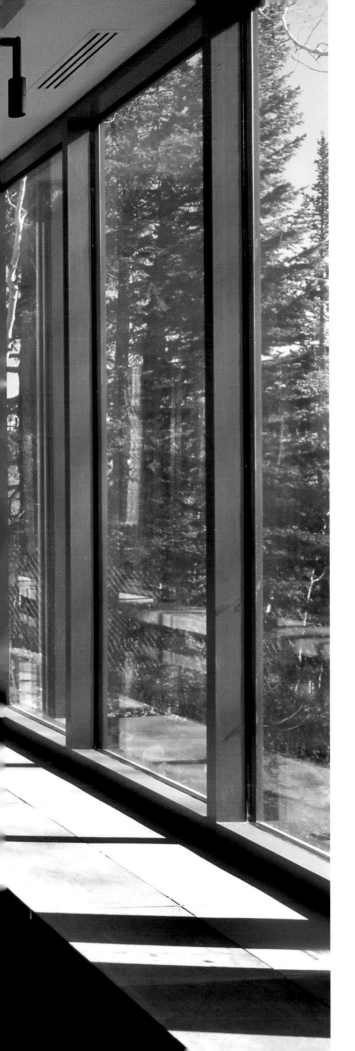

contents

TODAY HOME IS more than merely where the heart is. Home is more likely to be the heart of your fitness efforts—which, in turn, could be good for your heart, your mind, and your health in general.

There are several reasons for a heightened focus on home fitness, possibly the most urgent being the expansion of the waistline, particularly in America, where the national epidemic of obesity and the growing awareness of its detrimental health consequences are prompting a more proactive approach to health.

Those inclined to think that describing America's weight problem as an "epidemic" is an exaggeration may want to think again. And while they're thinking, they may want to get on the treadmill. According to a recent National Health and Nutrition Examination Survey, nearly two-thirds of the adults in the United States are overweight and 30.5 percent are obese, putting them at increased risk for diabetes, heart disease, stroke, hypertension, osteoporosis, sleep apnea, breathing problems, and some forms of cancer.

Defining the Problem

How did one nation arrive at this weighty predicament? Part of the problem is that technology has helped make life so much easier that most people need to burn off fewer calories during the course of the day. Most people drive rather than walk, take the elevator rather than climb stairs, sit at a desk all day rather than work in the fields, and watch TV for their evening recreation, rather than, let's say, go dancing. Yet for most people, food is plentiful—with the average diet excessively high in fat and calories.

A study by the Centers for Disease Control and Prevention found that one in four Americans gets virtually no exercise at all. Federal government guidelines recommend that Americans do at least 30 minutes of physical activity most days of the week. Reducing 100 calories per day or adding one half hour of exercise—such as a brisk walk—could go far in helping to eliminate the obesity epidemic.

Adding a little exercise to your day could also be good for your state of mind. Research by the Beckman Institute for Advanced Science and Technology at the University of Illinois shows that walking three times a week for 45 minutes not only significantly raised the walkers' heart rates but improved their ability to focus, an ability that seems to decline with age.

Fitting in Fitness

But what in the world does this lack of fitness phenomenon have to do with architecture and design? Well, successfully incorporating fitness into busy on-the-go lives means that exercise has to be more than convenient. It's easier to devote twenty minutes "here and there" to exercise if you don't also have to spend time going "there." If fitness is as easy as rolling out of bed and into the pool, you may actually swim a few laps on a regular basis.

As one way of meeting ever-more-hectic schedules, where there is no time to relegate to exercise per se, according to architects and designers, exercise areas have become a common request in homes of all sizes, with as many as one in five new luxury homes now featuring a gym. To fill these spaces, the National Sporting Goods Association says Americans spent $4.7 billion on exercise equipment in 2003, an increase of eight percent from the previous year, with treadmills being the most popular equipment.

Reshaping the home to accommodate fitness can be a simple or complex transformation, a low-maintenance endeavor or a high-tech operation. Fitness space can be as basic as turning a walk-in closet into a niche for a treadmill, as adaptable as fitting a dance studio into a New York City apartment, as comprehensive as planning for a two-story his-and-hers gym, or as organic as building a home exterior you can literally climb. Some traditional homes also serve as a flexible fitness center for the growing family, incorporating various forms of exercise into their changing priorities.

A growing number of new homes accord fitness so highly they have factored in a significant percentage of the floor space for exercise. As a rule, exercise rooms are getting larger—averaging 14 by 14 feet, the size of a secondary bedroom. To reframe the importance of fitness, layouts have given the workout room a new prominence, placing such rooms in a strategic location usually accorded to the living room; in the room with the best light or view; or in a room at the entrance to the home.

But even more visionary is the subtle concept of designing the whole home so that people are encouraged and even enticed into walking and moving more during the course of their regular activities throughout the day. Through such innovative features as stairs so appealing that they invite the viewer to climb them and elongated layouts that subtly add just a few more healthy steps to everyday activities, homeowners may find themselves exercising more without even knowing it. Forward-thinking architects have found new ways to painlessly fuse in fitness and interior designers are making workout paraphernalia more visually appealing. Fitness has become a stylish design element and is shaping a sleek, clean aesthetic.

All the evidence says it's time to get moving and, while you're at it, you may want to build the lean look of fitness into your home.

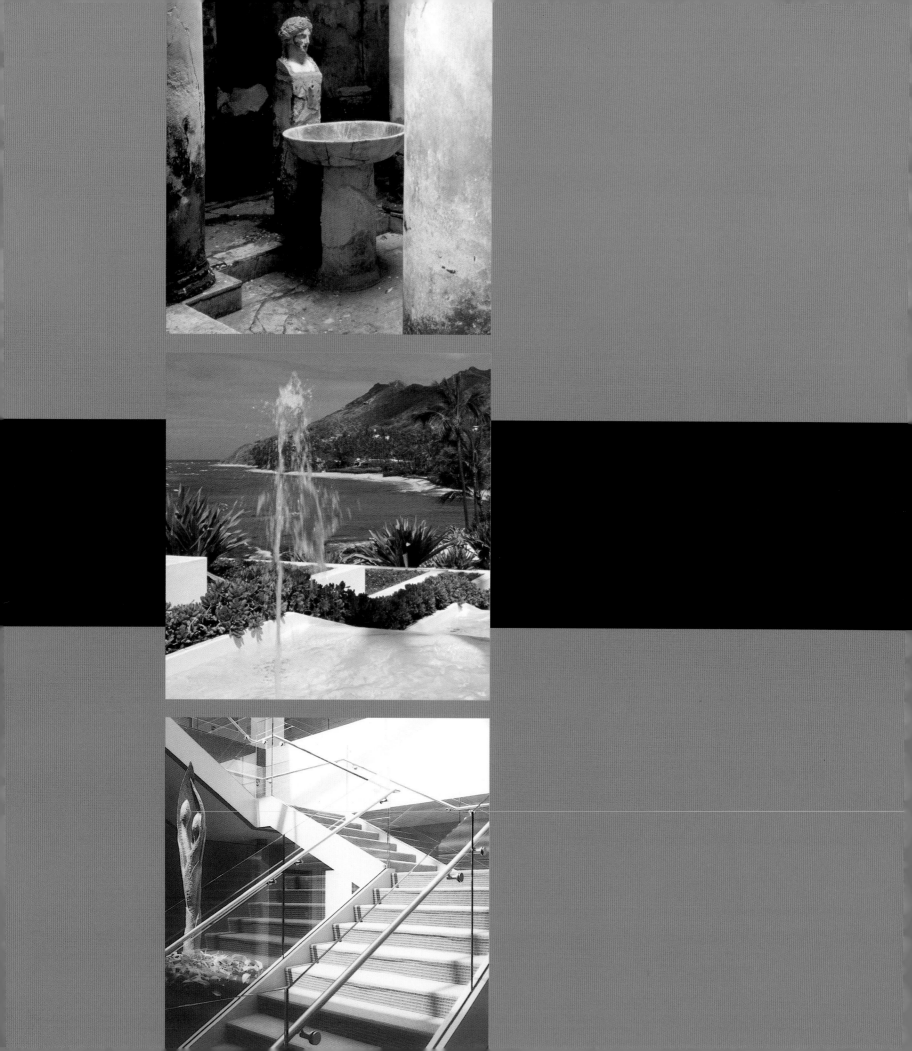

history

Exercise: Ancients and Moderns

ALTHOUGH PHYSICAL ACTIVITY has always sculpted the human body, it has not always shaped architecture. The importance of perfecting the human body—and creating buildings dedicated to that purpose—was well appreciated by the ancient Greeks. The word gym derives from the Greek word for "naked," *gymnos*, because physical competitions were usually performed outdoors without clothing.

Greek athletes attained celebrity status similar to that granted to athletes today. To encourage their efforts at self-perfection, the Greeks built various gymnasia devoted to different kinds of exercise. A gymnasium included a stadium, baths, covered porticos for practice in bad weather, plus a place for lectures. Gymnasia were primarily reserved for men. Greek women—except for Spartan women whose fitness was encouraged so they would become mothers of warriors—had to content themselves with daily walks in the inner courtyards of their homes.

In general, the Romans did not share the Greek enthusiasm for gymnastics training, but they did build baths of varying sizes, known as *thermae*. Similar to modern health clubs, these *thermae* contained shops, restaurants, exercise yards, libraries, and reading rooms or gymnasia centered around spacious gardens. Leaders of the Roman Empire built similar baths throughout its vast territories. Perhaps

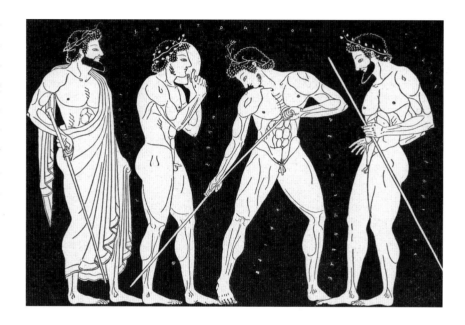

ABOVE: By the fourth and fifth century B.C., the ancient Greek Olympic games included such events as running, boxing, and wrestling, some of which were performed without the encumbrance of togas. Winners were honored with prizes and crowned with olive leaves, often their only adornment.

RIGHT: Large Roman baths or *thermae*, such as this one in Herculaneum, served as community centers for sports and recreation. The Romans established *thermae* in the far reaches of their empire and many ruins of these community centers remain today.

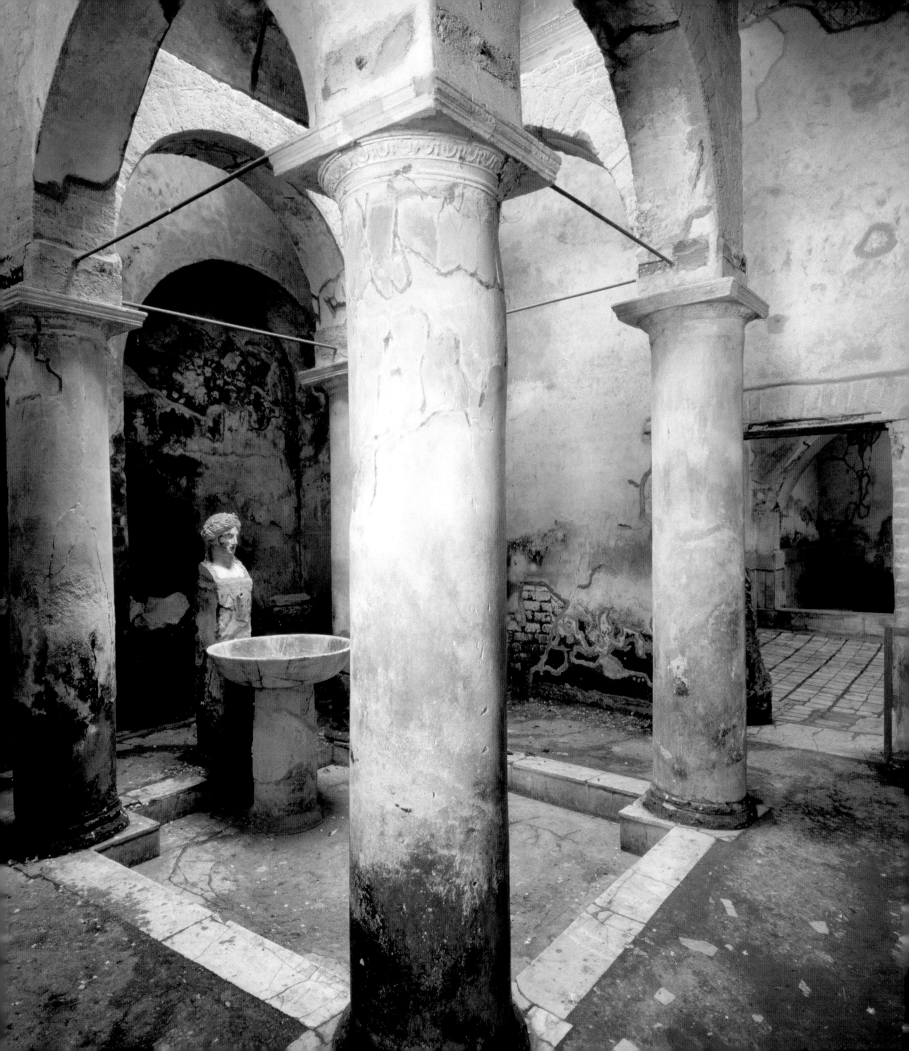

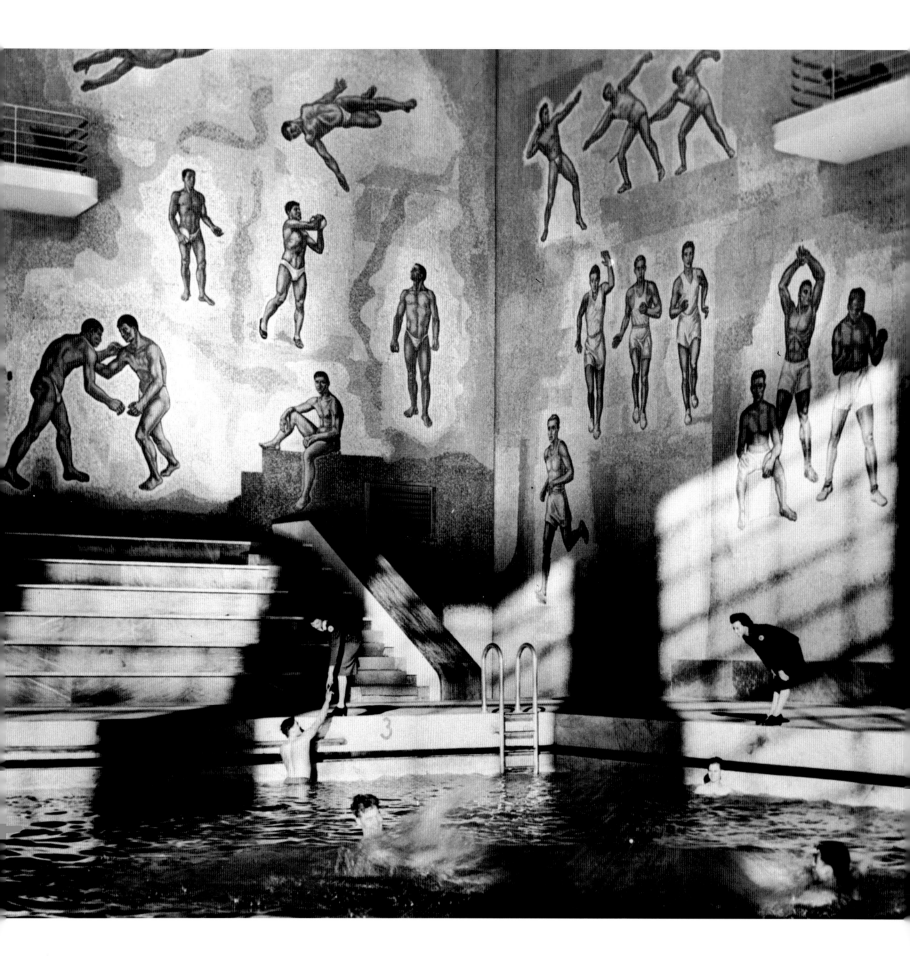

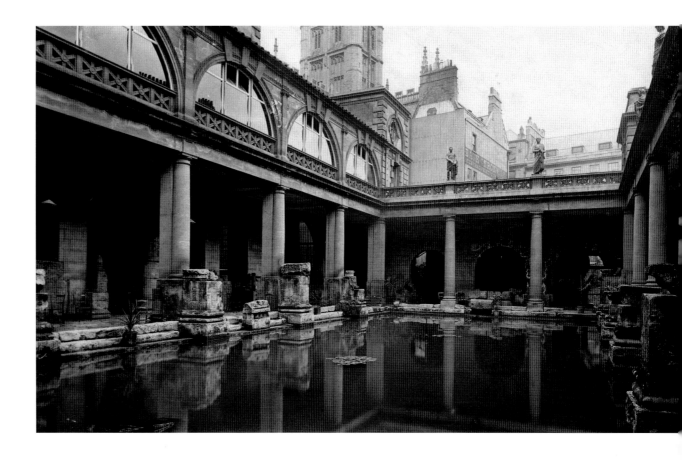

LEFT: The spirit of the ancient Olympics is evoked by these pool frescoes in the Foro Italica sports complex built by dictator Benito Mussolini. Here, Allied soldiers test the waters shortly after World War II. ABOVE RIGHT: Roman invaders between the first and fourth century AD built the remarkable bathhouses on the site of ancient Celtic hot springs located in the city of Bath, England. Bath's reputation as a fashionable spa town enjoyed a revival in the early 18th century when some of the ruins' original grandeur was restored.

the most famous to survive were those in Bath, England, which provided a fashionable resort even through Jane Austen's day.

After the fall of Rome, it would be centuries before physical fitness was a subject that excited enough interest to inspire any kind of construction. During the Middle Ages, the wealthy rode and hunted, but the average person worked long days of hard, physical labor and had no need for any additional exercise.

The Fitness Revival

The Renaissance revived interest in Greek ideals, which led to a desire to revive the Olympics. That movement climaxed in the mid-19th century in several fitness festivals featuring archery, gymnastics, cricket, fencing, rowing, jumping, running, soccer, and sailing. For centuries, physical fitness would remain focused on excelling in individual sports.

Before the modern Olympic Games officially reopened in 1896, interest in physical fitness had inspired the first public gym in Paris, opened by Hippolyte Triat, a vaudevillian strong man.

A 19th-century movement called "muscular Christianity" proposed physical fitness as a way to promote moral good and intellectual development. The idea was promoted by Sir George Williams, who in 1841 created the Young Men's Christian Association in London and exported the concept to the United States. Stateside, YMCAs encouraged fitness and supported collegiate sports. Swimming was taught there, basketball was invented there, and volleyball was created by a YMCA college graduate. After World War I, a stronger emphasis on physical education prompted more high schools to build gymnasiums.

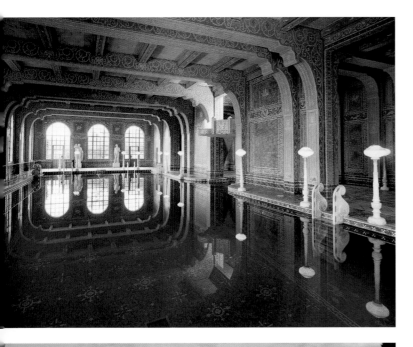

Fitness for the Privileged Few

During the 1920s and 30s the most famous examples of fitness in architecture in the United States, were the lavish pools, squash, and tennis courts that belonged to movie stars and millionaires such as William Randolph Hearst and Doris Duke. Hearst built two pools at his San Simeon estate. The indoor Roman Pool, built under Hearst's tennis courts, was inspired by an ancient Roman bath. It was lavishly lined with one-inch-square Murano mosaic tiles of glass and twenty-two-carat gold. The dazzling outdoor Neptune Pool features a Roman temple made with fragments of ancient columns and statues of Neptune and the Nereids.

Between 1936 and 1938, the American heiress and philanthropist Doris Duke built Shangri-La, her 14,000-square-foot Honolulu home and Islamic-style retreat, around a central patio open to the sky. It was designed by an architectural firm in New Delhi. Furnished with art, furniture, and architectural elements from Iran, Morocco, Turkey, Spain, Syria, Egypt, and India, the main house and its playhouse, with a central recreational room, are separated by a 75-foot swimming pool, water terraces, and steps of white marble. The landscape blends an Indian Mughal garden and water features with tropical gardens and breathtaking views of the Pacific Ocean.

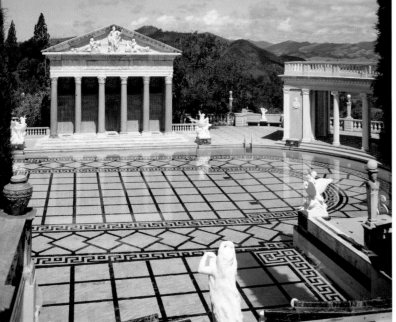

ABOVE LEFT: The indoor Roman Pool at Hearst's Castle was styled after the baths of Caracalla, built in Rome between 211 and 217 AD. The dazzling blue pool is decorated with glass tiles called *smalti*.
BELOW LEFT: It took twelve years for newspaper magnate W.R. Hearst to build San Simeon's outdoor Neptune Pool, which extends 104 feet long and is 58 feet wide.
RIGHT: Philanthropist Doris Duke built Shangri-La, her home and Islamic-style retreat, on five glorious acres of Hawaiian waterfront property. The landscaping around the 75-foot swimming pool blends an Indian Mughal garden, tropical gardens, and vistas of Diamond Head and the Pacific Ocean.

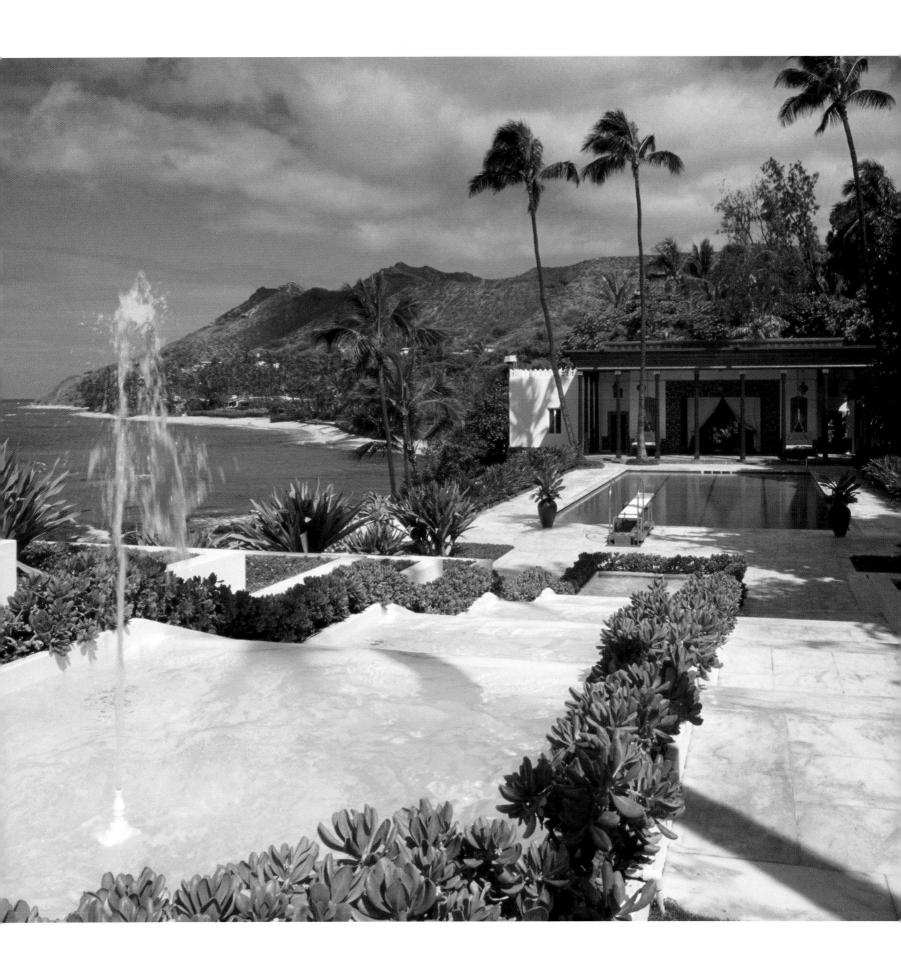

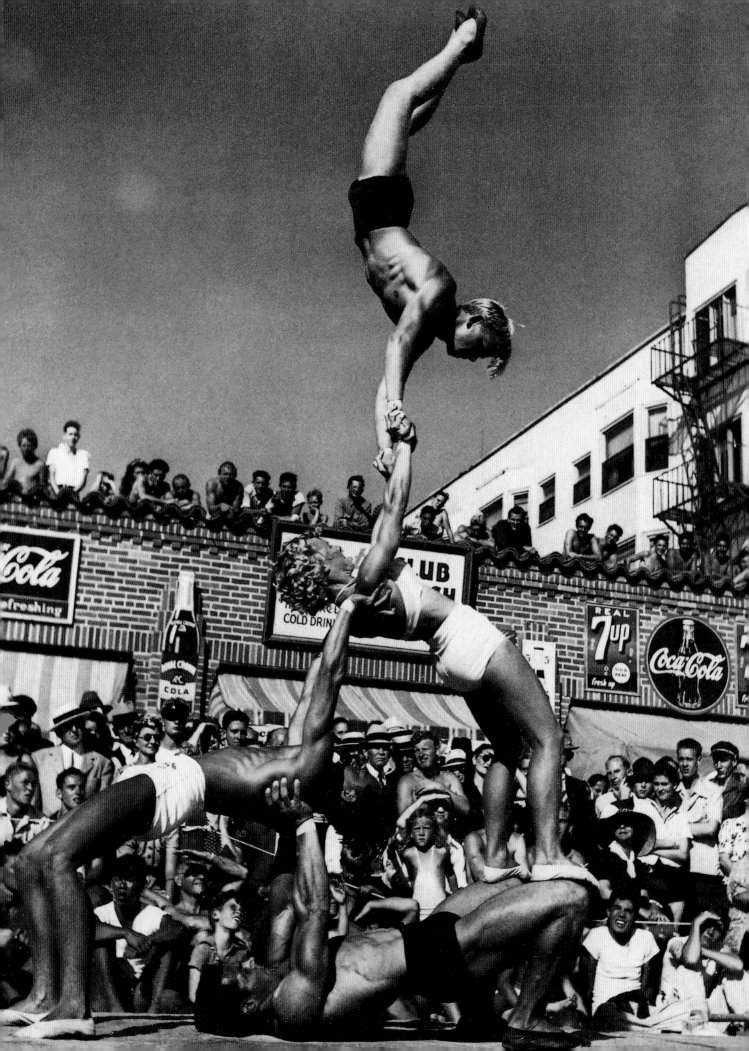

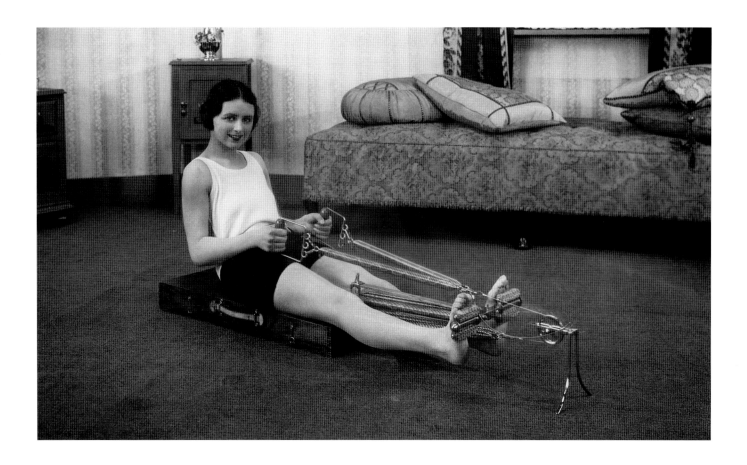

LEFT: This display of acrobatics was typical of the daring pyramids and other human constructions that drew crowds to Muscle Beach in Santa Monica, California, says Glenn "Whitey" Sundby, pictured here atop the pyramid. Sundby helps preserve Muscle Beach memories as president of the International Gymnastics Hall of Fame. ABOVE: Fortunately, home exercise equipment has come a long way since this precarious contraption was used to trim and tone thighs.

Muscle Culture

During the 1930s, 40s, and 50s, acrobats and bodybuilders helped create a California neighborhood when they gathered to demonstrate their strength and agility at a Santa Monica beach, renamed "Muscle Beach." The scene eventually moved to Venice, California, but many of the area regulars—Vic Tanney, Jack LaLanne, and Joe Gold—went on to become household names in fitness, building national chain-location gyms. Some regulars, such as Steve "Hercules" Reeves, became movie stars and stunt men, while others helped train the armed forces in World War II.

In 1956, the President's Council on Physical Fitness was created during the Dwight Eisenhower administration and promoted by John F. Kennedy, who wrote that his less-than-fit compatriots, "look instead of play; we ride instead of walk." Perhaps inspired by this admonition, Dr. Kenneth Cooper wrote about the importance of aerobic exercise in the late 1960s and helped boost a fitness movement that would eventually place gyms in hotels, cruise ships, college campuses, and corporate headquarters.

Muscle Culture Meets Car Culture

However, as the nation concerned itself with ways to become more fit, the negative effects of car culture had already taken their toll and would further deprive people of the basic exercise benefits gained from walking. At the start of the 20th century, there were fewer than 8,000 cars in the United States. By the 1960s, there were approximately 50,000; today there are almost 200 million. As car ownership increased, it shaped city planning, unfurling development into suburban sprawl and, many say, creating "waistline sprawl."

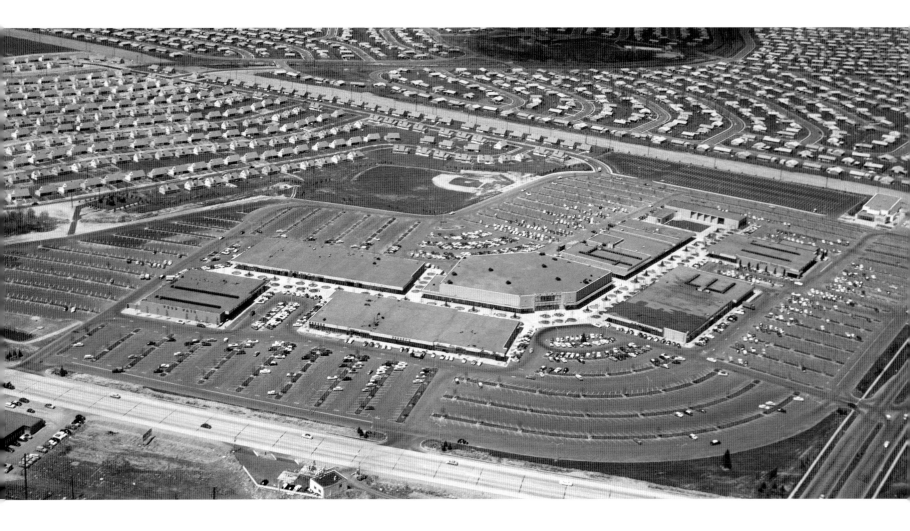

Soldiers returning home after World War II used the GI Bill to buy homes in suburban communities built for commuters with cars. Levittown, Long Island, was one of the first. Although built for commuters, it still retained a "village" feel. It had seven "greens" with stores, libraries, and swimming pools to which stay-at-home, carless housewives could walk, plus to which school children could ride their bikes. As the number of cars grew with families owning more than one car, more suburban developments were built without sidewalks or easy access to schools and commercial areas.

In sprawling suburbia, people had less motivation to walk during the course of the day. Buying a carton of milk required getting into the car. To get children to school, someone had to drive them. Could living up to the American dream of buying a home in the suburbs have made families flabbier?

"You buy a home as big as you want, you drive everywhere you want, and then you have kids that play Nintendo instead of basketball, that know three or four software programs instead of being able to run three miles," said Mark Dessauer, communications director of Active Living By Design, a national program of the Robert Wood Johnson Foundation, which evaluates approaches to increasing physical fitness through community design. Its September 2003 study, *Relationship Between Urban Sprawl and Physical Activity, Obesity, and Morbidity*—conducted

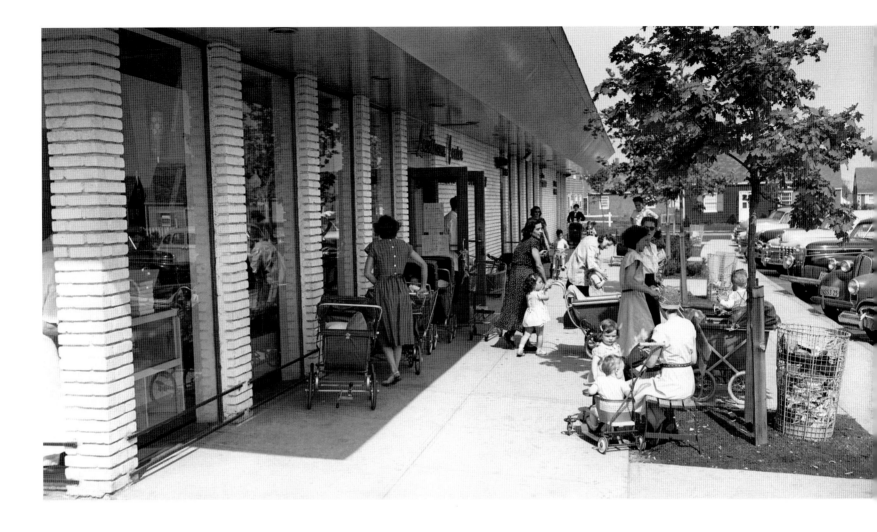

LEFT and RIGHT: The suburban community of Levittown was originally planned so that housewives who remained home during the day—without access to the family car—could still walk to stores and schools and socialize at pools or parks. As more families acquired a second car, suburban planning began to eliminate sidewalks and sprawl out in ways that defied the healthy exercise and social interaction inherent in walking.

for the National Center for Smart Growth, University of Maryland and supported by the Robert Wood Johnson Foundation, analyzed health data of 200,000 people living in 448 U.S. counties in major metropolitan areas. The study showed that as sprawl—the degree of spread between homes, shops, restaurants, and other destinations—increases so do the chances that residents will be obese or have high blood pressure. People living in sprawling counties are likely to walk less, and whether or not they participate in a form of physical activity, the simple act of walking during the day can make a difference. Curbing suburban sprawl in favor of compact, walkable communities will become an important strategy for curbing waistline sprawl.

New Urbanism

To foster healthier communities, many city planners now know that they have to create walk-to destinations. The urban design movement known as New Urbanism, which began in the late 1980s, focuses on the importance of building neighborhoods in which a person can meet his or her daily needs within a five-minute walk. One way to accomplish this is to mix commercial and residential space. Another is to factor in wider, more navigable sidewalks and, in some cases, create sidewalks where none existed. Placing speed bumps in streets makes them safer for bike riders. Communities with a focus on physical health might be built around recreational facilities, and include walking or

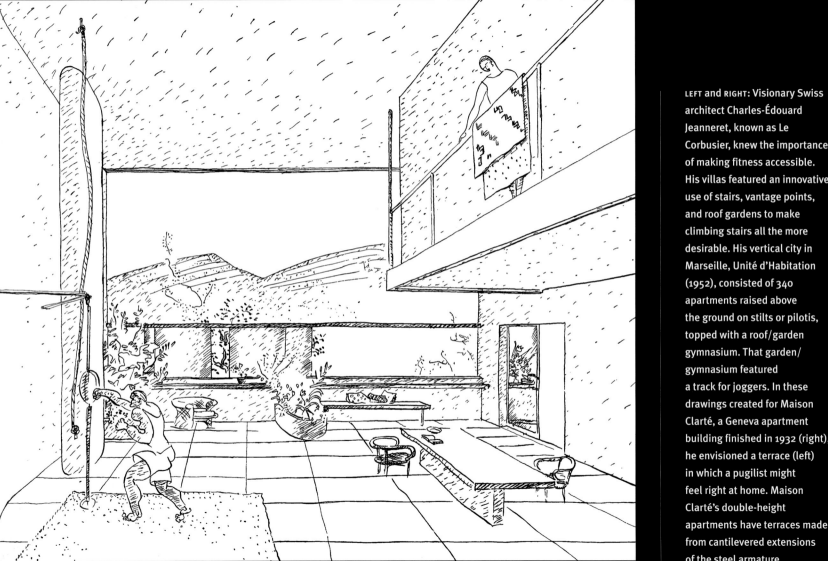

LEFT and **RIGHT:** Visionary Swiss architect Charles-Édouard Jeanneret, known as Le Corbusier, knew the importance of making fitness accessible. His villas featured an innovative use of stairs, vantage points, and roof gardens to make climbing stairs all the more desirable. His vertical city in Marseille, Unité d'Habitation (1952), consisted of 340 apartments raised above the ground on stilts or pilotis, topped with a roof/garden gymnasium. That garden/gymnasium featured a track for joggers. In these drawings created for Maison Clarté, a Geneva apartment building finished in 1932 (right), he envisioned a terrace (left) in which a pugilist might feel right at home. Maison Clarté's double-height apartments have terraces made from cantilevered extensions of the steel armature.

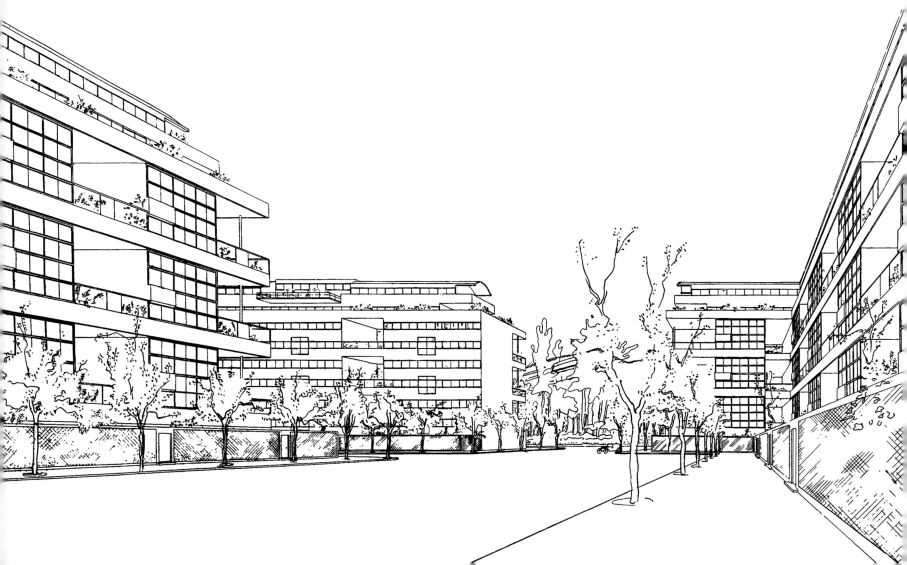

jogging trails for adults, play areas for children, and/or a fitness center.

These concepts have also gained recognition in the planning of corporate buildings as companies explore ways to increase worker productivity and reduce health-care costs.

Healthier Corporate Buildings

While planning the renovation and expansion of the Robert Wood Johnson Foundation's New Jersey facility in the mid-1990s, Phil Dordai, a principal of the Princeton-based Hillier Architecture, talked with his clients about how the incidence of obesity and the declining amount of daily activity could be addressed by building design.

"The standard developer model by default always makes travel distances from the parking lot to the front door as short as possible," said Dordai. "We began to realize that this was the wrong answer. The real answer should be that maybe you should make people get up and walk, create destinations that people want to go to other than their specific work stations. Make them get up and move during the course of the day."

Completed in 2002, the foundation's two-story building includes a mall-like atrium with a library, coffee bar, and meeting place. There is a dining area at one end and an auditorium at the other. Aggregating activities in this way creates a desirable destination; putting them on an outside wall with natural light makes it even more attractive. Stairs can become a StairMaster if they are attractive enough. Stairwells can be widened to encourage climbing and artwork

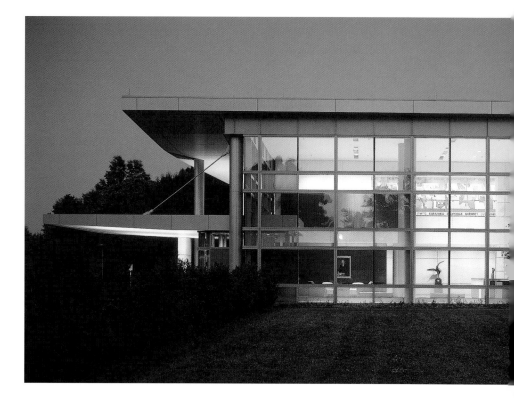

might be hung there to attract interest. Fire stairs can be positioned so they are convenient and the doors left open so people are more likely to use them.

"You have to counteract the computer couch potato problem. The whole world comes to you via your computer so you don't have to get up and talk to anyone. If you've grown up that way, it's even more so the case," said Dordai. "We felt we had to create places within the building that people would want to go."

Creating a campus of buildings, rather than expanding vertically, makes it easier to encourage walking and jogging outside. In Sprint's new 200-acre headquarters in Overland Park, Kansas, also designed by Hillier, parking garages are a five-minute walk, which is more than the 150-foot distance consid-

ABOVE: The New Jersey office of the Robert Wood Johnson Foundation is designed to encourage more walking by employees. Destinations for communal activities, such as a coffee bar and meeting room, are aggregated at a desirable distance. **RIGHT, ABOVE and BELOW:** The building's designers, Princeton-based Hillier Architecture widened and brightly lit the stairs, displaying art work along the wall to draw the eye— and eventually the rest of the body—up the stairs.

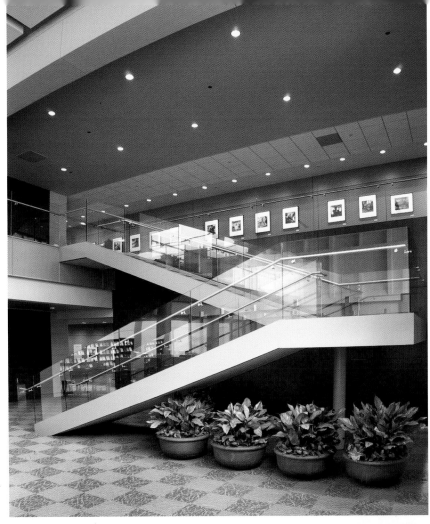

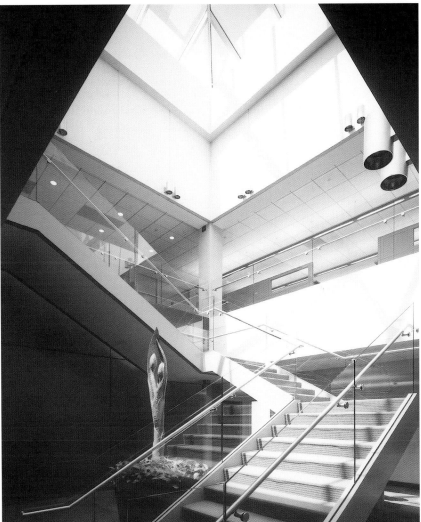

ered standard. Although there was space to build four smaller parking lots, only one central lot was created, making sure all employees would walk at least a few minutes each day.

Designed to look like a college campus, the Sprint headquarters has five major courtyards with a fitness center, retail stores, cafés, and recreation areas. There are outdoor walking paths with flowers and fountains. Instead of being designed around the car, the campus is planned around the pedestrian. Since the buildings are only four stories tall, and the elevators are designed to be less attractive than the stairs, employees are encouraged to climb.

"We should design buildings and communities that encourage people to be more physically active," said Dordai. "At the residential level that should be solved at the level of planning. Too much new development is being designed without sidewalks and uses land inefficiently, discouraging people from walking."

How Technology Can Help

Although technology may share the blame for the sprawling waistline, it may also one day help create a healthier home. Scientists at MIT's Changing Places/Houses project are researching the way the home of the future may help encourage healthy behavior.

"Our vision is that technology can be used to get people information when they are receptive to it," said Stephen Intille, a research scientist with MIT's Department of Architecture and the technology director of Changing Places/Houses. "We are working on technologies that can be embedded into

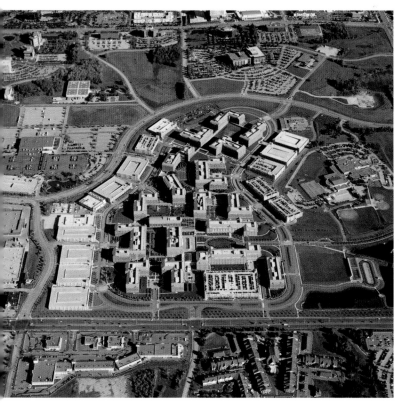

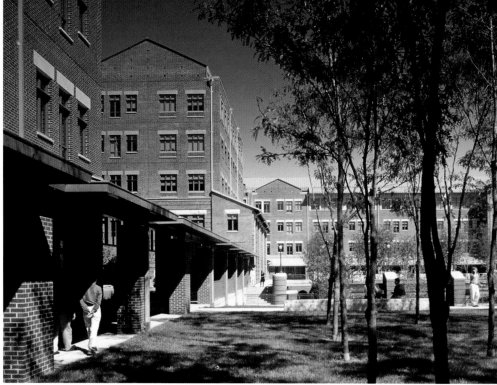

the environment and that can be used to motivate behavior changes."

A series of studies on stair use found that placing a sign about the health benefits of stair climbing at their base prompted more people to use them. Similarly, says Intille, a monitoring device such as a cell phone, your computer, or something embedded into the architecture of your home—working with motion sensors—could motivate you to exercise more, and reinforce your efforts by providing positive, personalized feedback.

For example, a sensor monitor can "guesstimate" how much exercise you get by walking during the course of one day so you would know if you reached the recommended amount. Homes might include interactive vir-

tual aerobics trainers (which already exist) built into the wall of a home gym. These trainers can sense how you move, provide corrections on a move, and even positive reinforcement, such as saying you did a "good job!"

Homes should definitely have more stairs, says Intille. In homes of the future, stairs should be "physically beautiful, a structural centerpiece that encourages you to climb them," but stairs can also provide entertaining ways to motivate movement. For example, the Soundstair exhibit, created by Christopher Janney and displayed in the Boston Museum of Science, uses the movement of feet on its steps to create music. As people move up and down the stairs their activity plays musical rhythms.

ABOVE, LEFT and RIGHT: Sprint's headquarters in Overland Park, Kansas was purposely designed in the manner of a campus. Only one parking lot was created so employees would have to walk to their buildings from a central location.

high fit home

"This little added piece of digital information makes climbing stairs a fun, game-like thing but in the process people are getting more exercise," said Intille.

A similar idea that might get children moving is to embed a digital system into the floor that works like the game Dance Dance Revolution, in which children must move their feet to different pads on a floor board. Or a new generation of video games could encourage children to move through the house.

Supplying a digital buddy might promote pedaling on a stationary bike. Many people don't like to exercise alone, so the home gym of the future might link a computer to an exercise bike. Not only could you look at virtual scenery while you ride, you could find a buddy online to bike with. If you get up at 6:30 A.M., say, and want cycling company, you could do an Internet search, find someone on the same schedule, and chat with them while you ride.

"First you create a physical design that encourages people to walk," said Intille, "then you add a digital system that makes it much more potentially entertaining."

As the importance of fitness becomes more apparent, some tools from the past—and some from the future—will help homes help their owners achieve their full fitness potential. Many of these are already in the works today—either on the drawing board, in experimental use, or incorporated into avant-garde commercial and residential environments.

BELOW LEFT: As hoped for, the additional steps added up and many employees lost some weight. BELOW RIGHT: The Sprint campus, also designed by Hillier Architecture, has five major courtyards with a fitness center, retail stores, cafés—and a recreation center—something for everyone to amble toward.

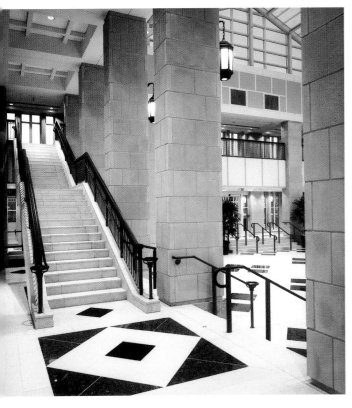

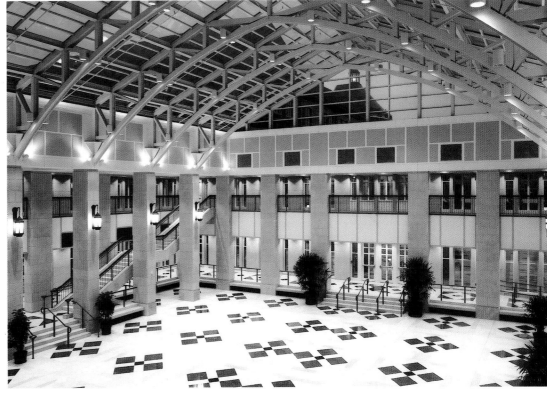

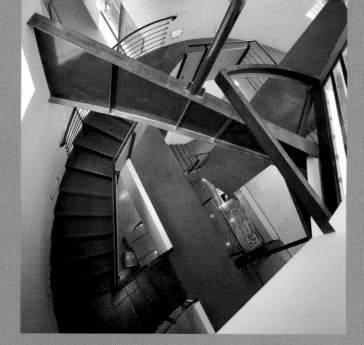

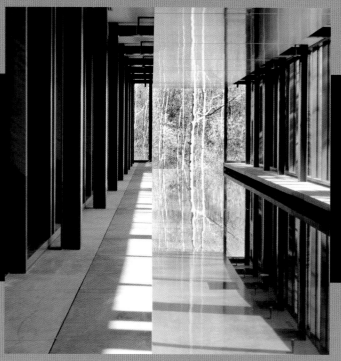

high

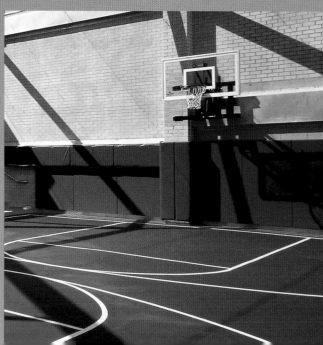

fit profiles

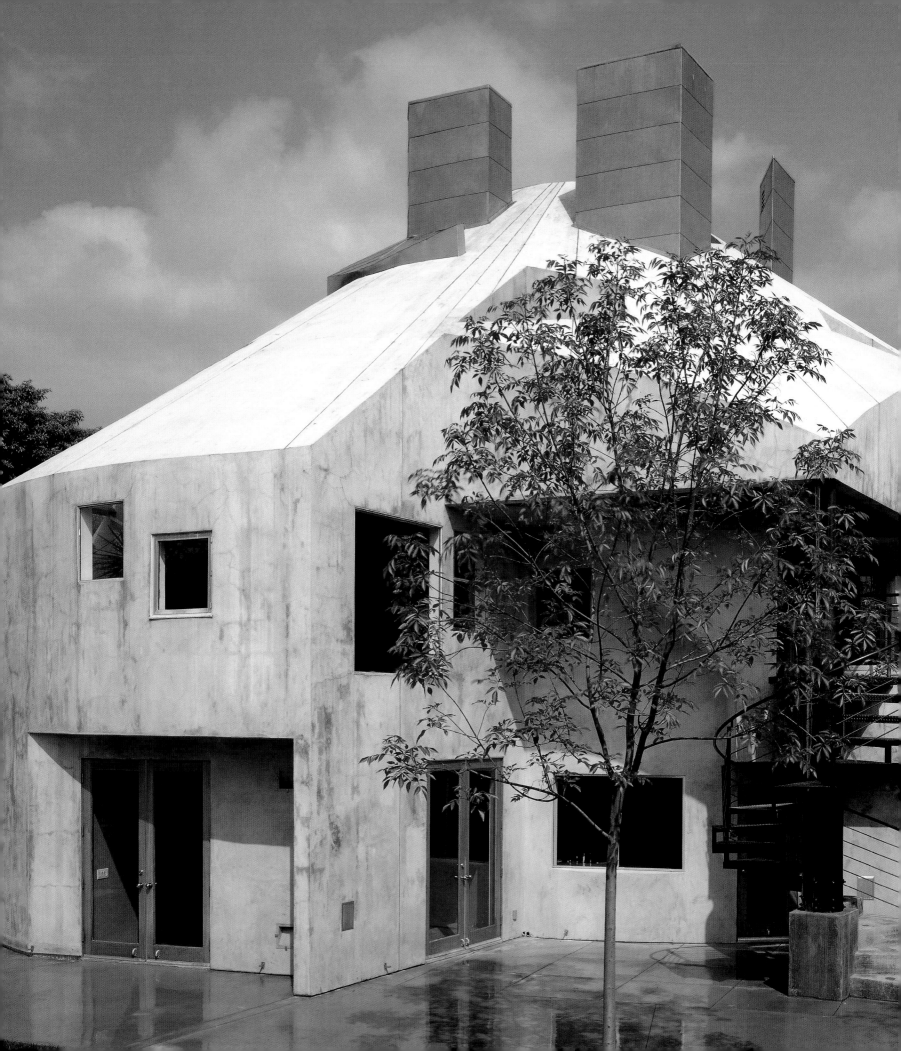

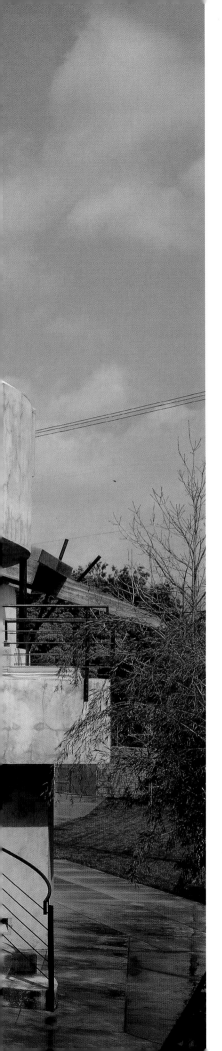

Inspiring Perpetual Motion

THE LAWSON/WESTEN HOUSE

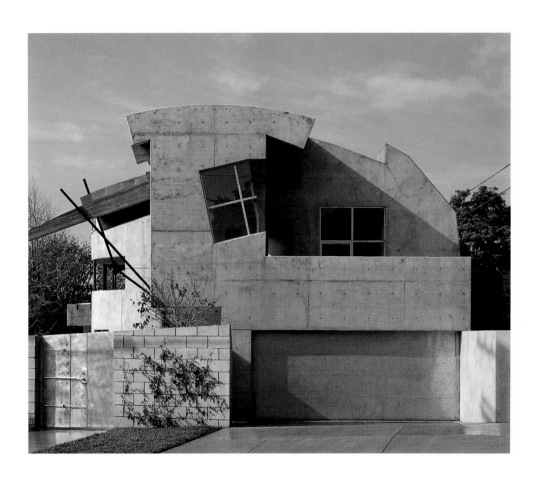

LEFT and **ABOVE:** The changing perspectives and quixotic directions of this home's design give concrete evidence to the notion that so much of beauty is motion.

AS THIS WEST LOS ANGELES HOUSE was built, its layout seemed to evolve and shift subtly, changing perspectives and vantage points but not priorities. The original scheme for the kitchen had three rectangular plan elements, the remnants of which now appear in various parts of the kitchen. The kitchen is where the homeowners spend much of their time, so it was the focal point of the design. But not all elements of that focal point were

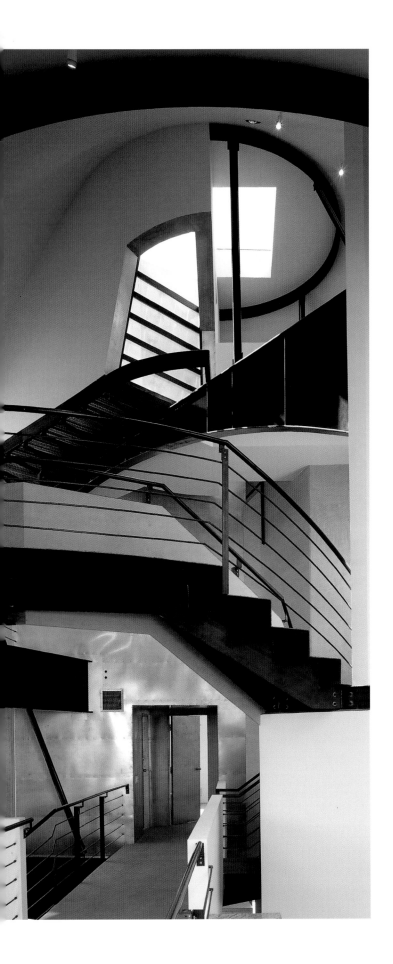

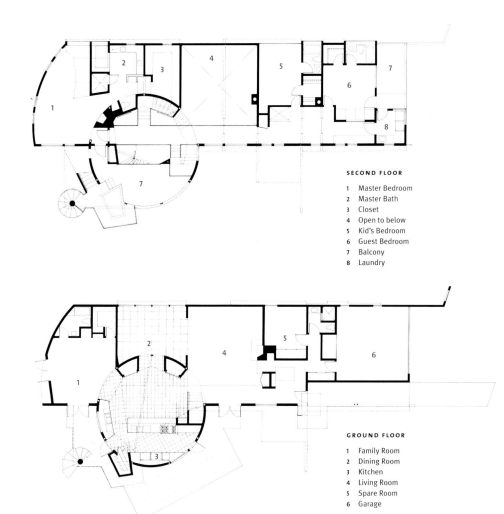

SECOND FLOOR

1 Master Bedroom
2 Master Bath
3 Closet
4 Open to below
5 Kid's Bedroom
6 Guest Bedroom
7 Balcony
8 Laundry

GROUND FLOOR

1 Family Room
2 Dining Room
3 Kitchen
4 Living Room
5 Spare Room
6 Garage

fixed, and the kitchen can now be seen from perspectives not originally imagined.

As the owners saw their home being built, they would ask, "Why is this piece of kitchen over here?" The answer was that the piece related to a scheme that was no longer there—things had shifted ever so subtly.

The plan of the kitchen—established a set of rules in an order that realigned as they were applied practically. As a result of the flexible interpretations of the dimensions, the house seems to encourage exploration by offering distinctive views at varying levels of the same rooms.

LEFT: The stairs in this home seem to spiral and soar like double helix strands of DNA. An abundance of natural light and interposed galleries make the ascent an experience to savor. RIGHT: Each lyrical gallery, reached by yet a few more steps, invites a serenade.

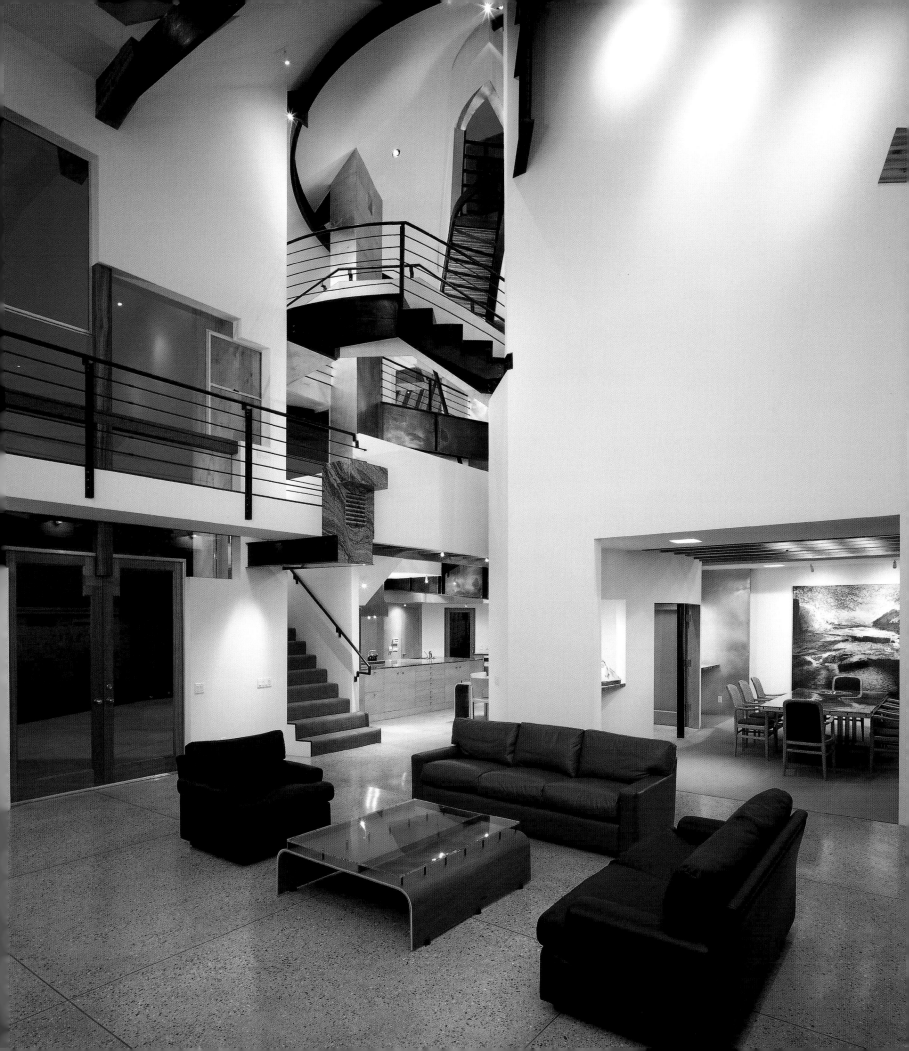

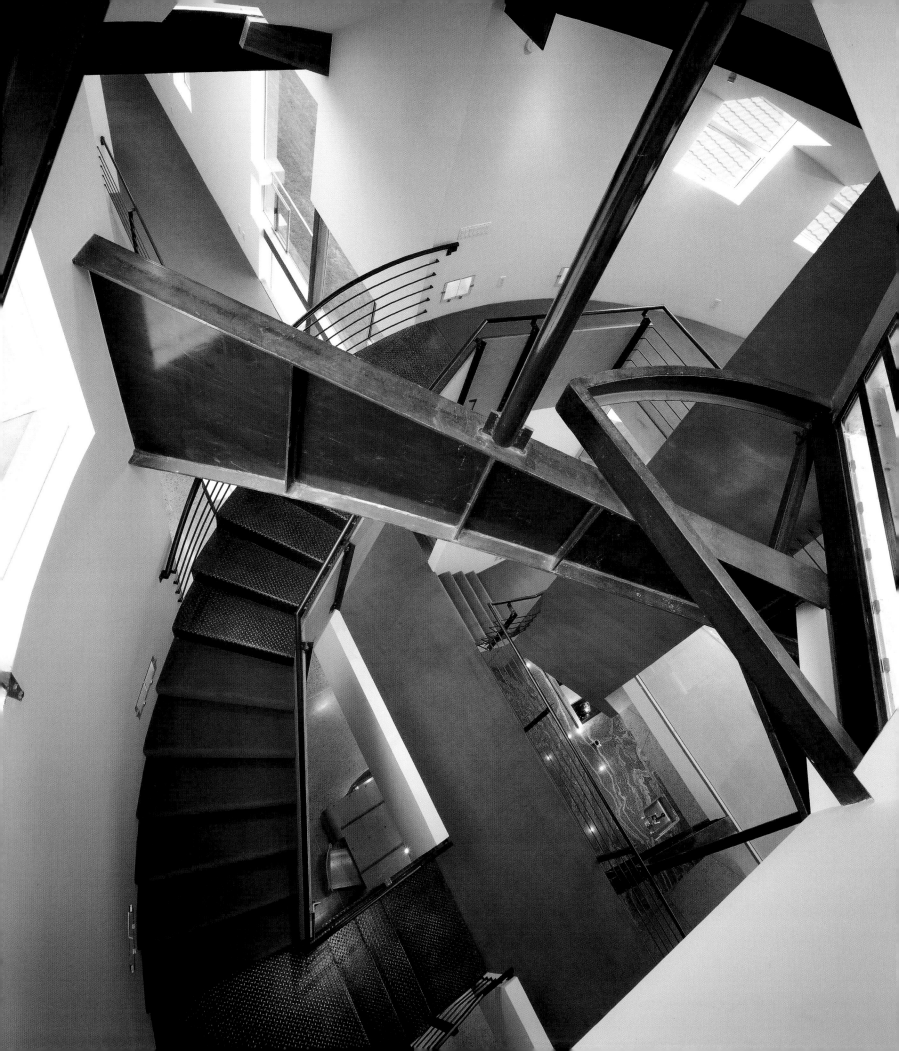

The house testifies happily to all the interesting things an architect can do with stairs. Imaginative configurations create balconies and viewing platforms whimsical enough to elicit serenades.

Stairs cut boldly across vast expanses of open space, with geometric extensions of the support system creating a visual counterpoint. The steps twist and turn in arcs and angles, as much art as conveyance. Distinctively shaped skylights, windows, and doors create intriguing light shapes as the sun shines through them.

The essential component of the house is a three-level hybrid cylindrical-conical volume that holds up the ground-floor kitchen. The cone becomes the roof shape of the cylindrical kitchen, but the center of the cone is not the center of the cylinder. The cone top is cut off, creating an ocean view deck. The cone is also sliced vertically, resulting in a parabolic curve. Pulling the curve toward the street lends rise to the vaulted roof.

Every step around or through the house changes its outlook and urges visitors to step further, pause a while, and continue.

LEFT: The stairs, which dissect and connect portions of this home can be seen as a form of sculpture. The climber not only exercises by ascending the stairs but adds a human dimension to the sculpture, exercising its true potential. RIGHT: Distinctively shaped skylights and doors offer fascinating patterns of light that also heighten the sensation of motion.

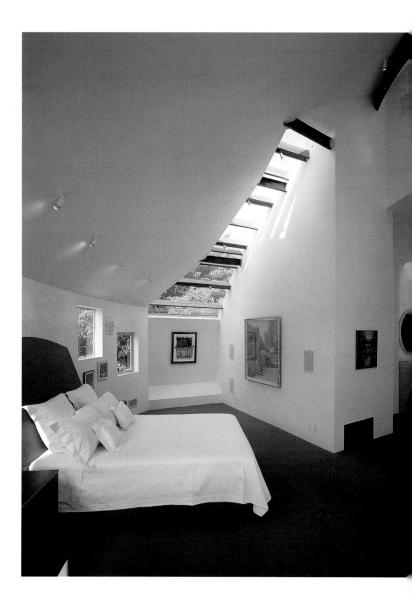

eric owen moss

Architectural Gymnastics at Play

THE ARONOFF GUESTHOUSE

THERE'S NO NEED for a StairMaster in this whimsical take on "the high-fit home" designed by Eric Owen Moss. As an architect Moss not only seeks to transform but also to keep architecture in a perpetual state of motion. This home is a prime example of how compelling such motion can be. It encourages stair climbing through its inventive orientation and inspired use of desirable vantage points.

This home makes climbing stairs seem like a winning game move. As quixotic as a Rubik's cube, was this guesthouse was designed to be a pleasurable toy for its owners and their employees, guests, and children. The building can be climbed on, examined, and used as a viewing platform.

The building is situated on the northern side of the Santa Monica Mountains on property that stretches down a slope to the Santa Monica Conservancy, a beautiful wooded area extending several miles and protected from development. The building's location

BELOW, LEFT and RIGHT: This idiosyncratic guesthouse embodies the architect's desire to keep architecture in a perpetual state of motion. The exterior has enough twists and turns to simulate a roller coaster ride. Inside, the guesthouse is all business; it contains a studio, an office, and an apartment.

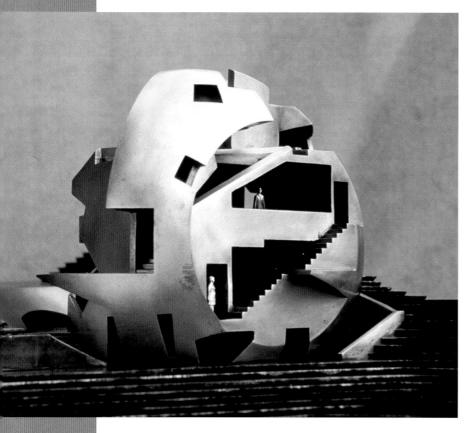

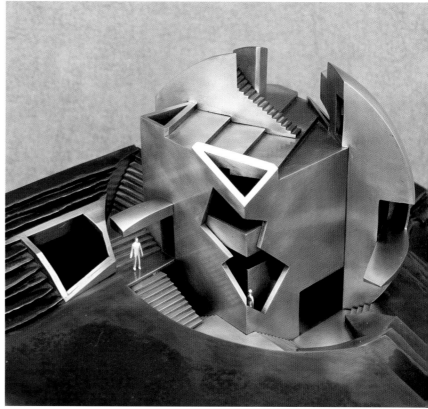

and the configuration of floors and windows maximize spectacular views of forest.

The guesthouse—which combines a studio, an office, and a private apartment—is located at the transition from the flat to the sloping portion of the site, exulting in its panoramic vantage point without interrupting views from the existing house. There are three floors to the guesthouse: the top-level studio/executive offices for the owners; an office floor at grade level for a business with three employees; and a separate apartment for an elderly father. The roof is designed as a stepped bleacher/deck with open and covered areas, oriented to the view of the Conservancy area and the San Fernando Valley. It is accessible from all levels via stairs that run along the perimeter of the house. It is also accessible internally, directly from the third floor.

The middle (grade) level is the office floor, used during the workday in conjunction with the owner's office on the top floor. The apartment at the lowest level has elevator access, a covered deck area, and an open patio. All levels are accessible from the middle level lobby or from the exterior.

Acknowledging a hillside profile, the guesthouse emerges from a conical cut dug at the side of the hill. It seems ready to tumble down the hill and invites exploration much the way a maze does.

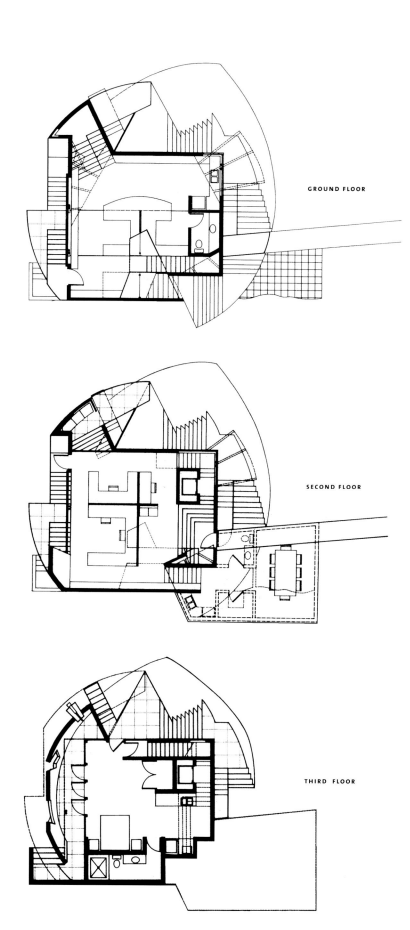

GROUND FLOOR

SECOND FLOOR

THIRD FLOOR

A Wing and a View

THE POOL HOUSE

IN THIS ETHEREAL EXTENSION of a Utah home, designed by Bohlin Cywinski Jackson, swimming can seem like soaring.

Already a dedicated swimmer, one of the home's owners has a new impetus to swim laps every day—to delight in the stunning views their swimming pool affords. The reflections inherent in the shimmering 25-meter pool wing seem to transport the swimmer through the forest landscape below—a 13-acre site densely covered with quaking aspens and thick firs, adjacent to nearby ski runs.

The pool seems to be in a physical realm unto itself, floating above surrounding trees and over a downhill stream of melting snow during the spring months. A band of stainless steel on the ceiling, which is the exact width of the pool, captures reflections on the ceiling, creating watery illusions, extending the view upward.

"As you swim toward the north end, the hillside is quite steep, and you are aware of the flowing stream below, as well as the extraordinary views. The short end of the pool looks out to the aspen forest, and the long view reflects from the pool surface and the stainless steel ceiling. You feel as if you're in a magic world," said Peter Bohlin, a principal with Bohlin Cywinski Jackson, a firm known for its ability to reflect both the nature of a home's place and the people who

RIGHT: In this home amidst the Utah Mountains, the 25-meter swimming pool has been awarded its own wing. With the wing's transparent walls, daily laps can lend the swimmer the illusion of soaring through the forest, into the mountains and over a trickling stream. This view of the pool wing glows with reflected light in the sylvan twilight.

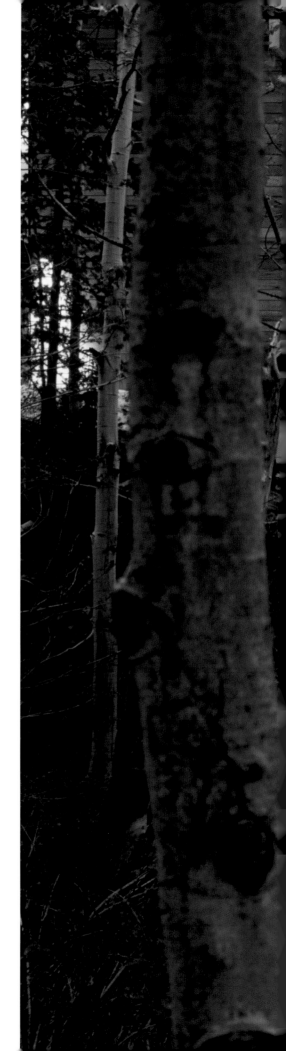

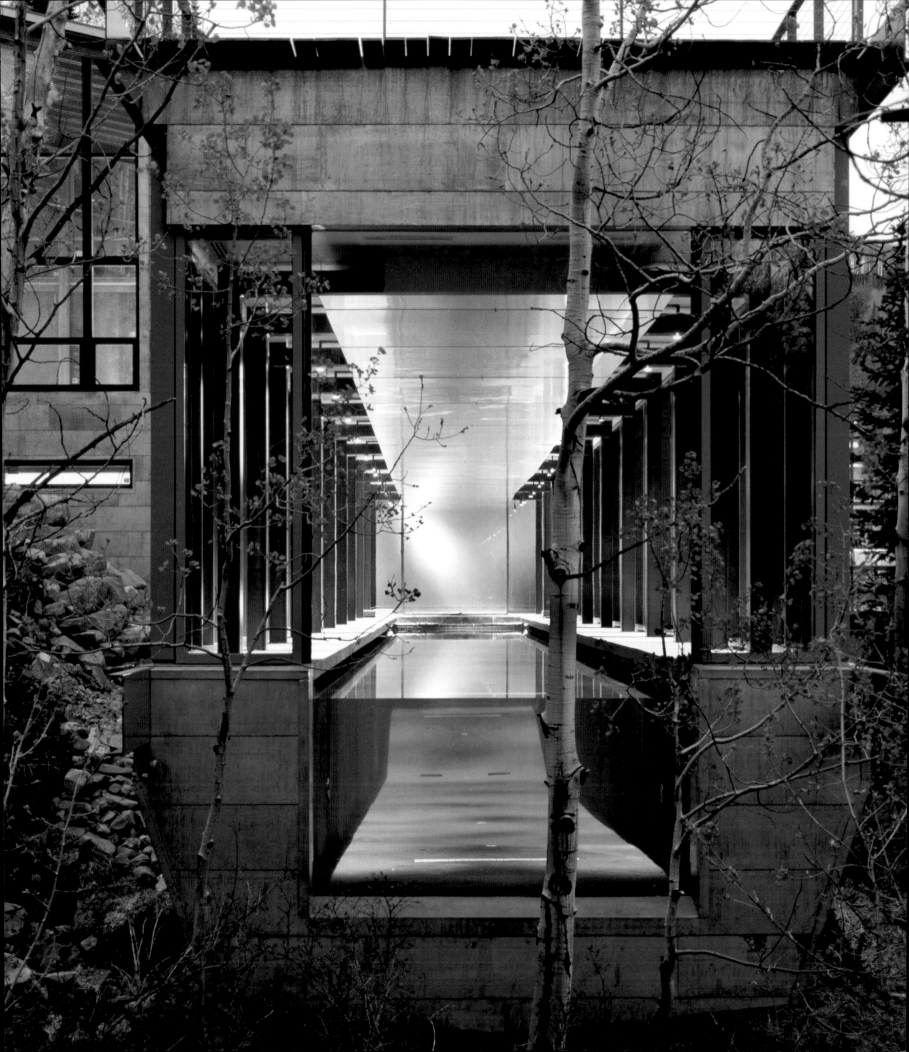

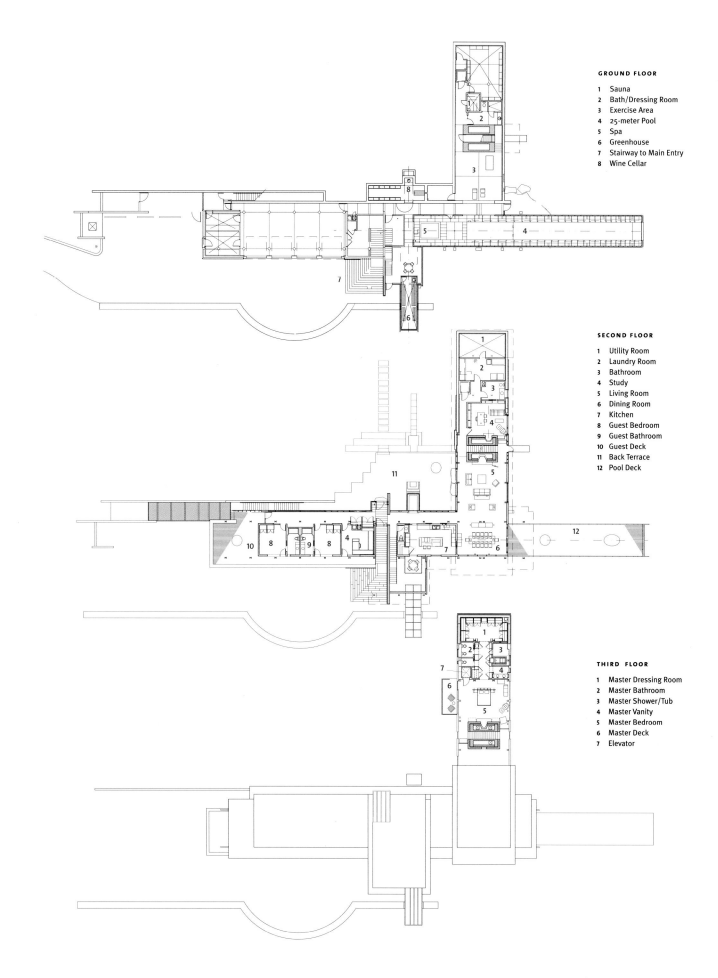

GROUND FLOOR

1 Sauna
2 Bath/Dressing Room
3 Exercise Area
4 25-meter Pool
5 Spa
6 Greenhouse
7 Stairway to Main Entry
8 Wine Cellar

SECOND FLOOR

1 Utility Room
2 Laundry Room
3 Bathroom
4 Study
5 Living Room
6 Dining Room
7 Kitchen
8 Guest Bedroom
9 Guest Bathroom
10 Guest Deck
11 Back Terrace
12 Pool Deck

THIRD FLOOR

1 Master Dressing Room
2 Master Bathroom
3 Master Shower/Tub
4 Master Vanity
5 Master Bedroom
6 Master Deck
7 Elevator

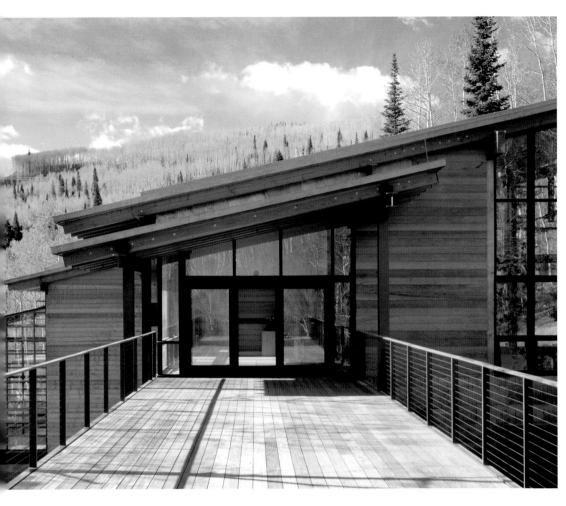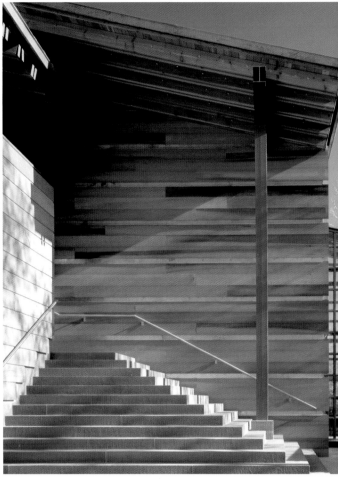

bohlin cywinski jackson

ABOVE LEFT: A deck covering the expanse of the pool wing, offers stunning views of the surrounding mountains that are similar to those enjoyed in the pool. The extensive use of natural materials such as Douglas fir is part of what helps the home fit so neatly into the landscape. ABOVE RIGHT: Cedar siding is used for cladding both interior and exterior walls and these crisply detailed stairs.

live there. "Creating a pool of this nature would inevitably stretch beyond the footprint of the house, so we took advantage of this extension to project out over the stream and to further intensify its relationship with the landscape," said Bohlin.

The 11,000-square-foot house is layered into the steep hillside with three different levels, the lowest occupying the most fitness space. Not only does the house fit neatly into the landscape but the materials used also complement the wooded nature of the site. Douglas fir is used throughout the roof structure and provides continuous warmth in the ceiling plane. The various heights of the roofs further define the intersecting spaces. Structural steel assemblies articulate connections between

roof, fireplace, and stair. Cedar siding is used for cladding both exterior and interior walls; thick, cast-in-place concrete walls convey the mass of the mountain beyond; glass allows a strong visual connection to the landscape.

The level from which the pool protrudes also includes a spa at one end of the pool, a greenhouse for growing orchids, and a sky-lit wine cellar. Adjacent to the pool are an exercise room, sauna, and bath/dressing area. Above the pool is the deck that extends from the dining area, with an expansive view almost identical to that from the pool. In this house, the pool and exercise floor has its own discrete entrance from the exterior at ground level.

The exercise room and the pool are separated by a glass wall, so when you are

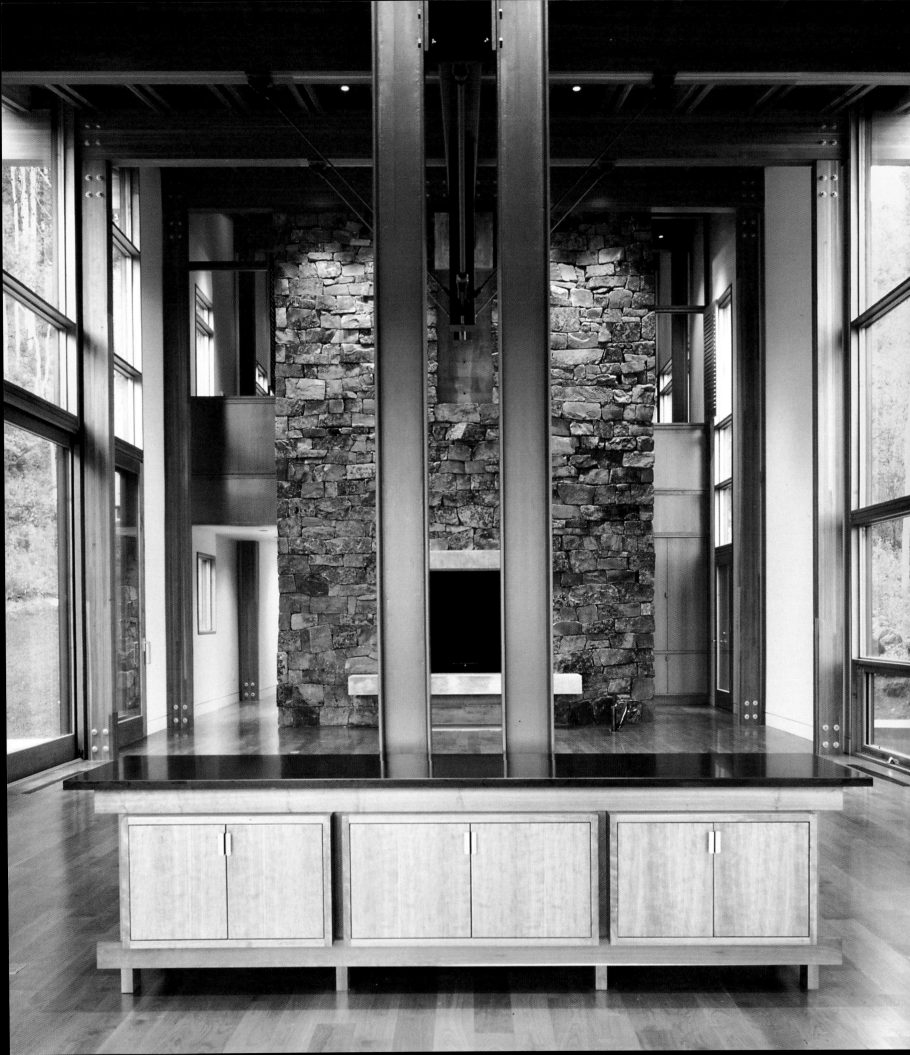

working out, you can look through the pool to the forest beyond. About one-quarter of the house is devoted to fitness. All the rooms on this level have something to do with revving up the body, reviving the spirit, and refreshing the mind.

"There's also a strong visual relationship between these rooms," said Bohlin. "A staircase threads down from the master bedroom through the living area to the exercise spaces. Through this stair, the pool is visible from the living and sleeping master bedrooms to which they are clearly connected."

According to Bohlin, any way in which you participate with the environment—hiking, walking, swimming, or climbing stairs—can be an emotionally satisfying and telling experience. Stairs may be considered an important and transformative part of the home's exercise equipment. Not only do they connect people to the exercise areas but they are, in a way, equivalent to one's experience of the pool, because climbing them and using them to move through the house can change people physically and emotionally.

"The whole business of getting from here to there is powerful stuff. It enables people and reveals the nature of the world to them," said Bohlin.

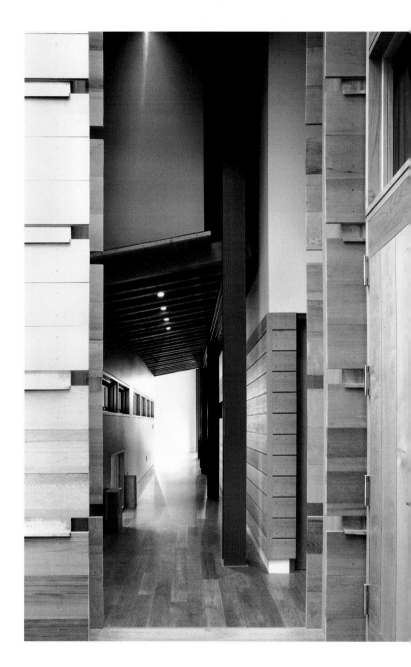

LEFT: About one-quarter of this home is devoted to fitness with the pool, a spa, and exercise room on the lower level. A staircase threads down from the master bedroom to the exercise spaces. Through the stair, the pool is visibly connected to the living room and the master bedroom. RIGHT: The hallways and stairs that connect the exercise and living spaces are considered a vital part of the home's exercise equipment. OVER: The highly reflective ceiling and glass walls of this lap pool wing add an ethereal visual element to daily exercise

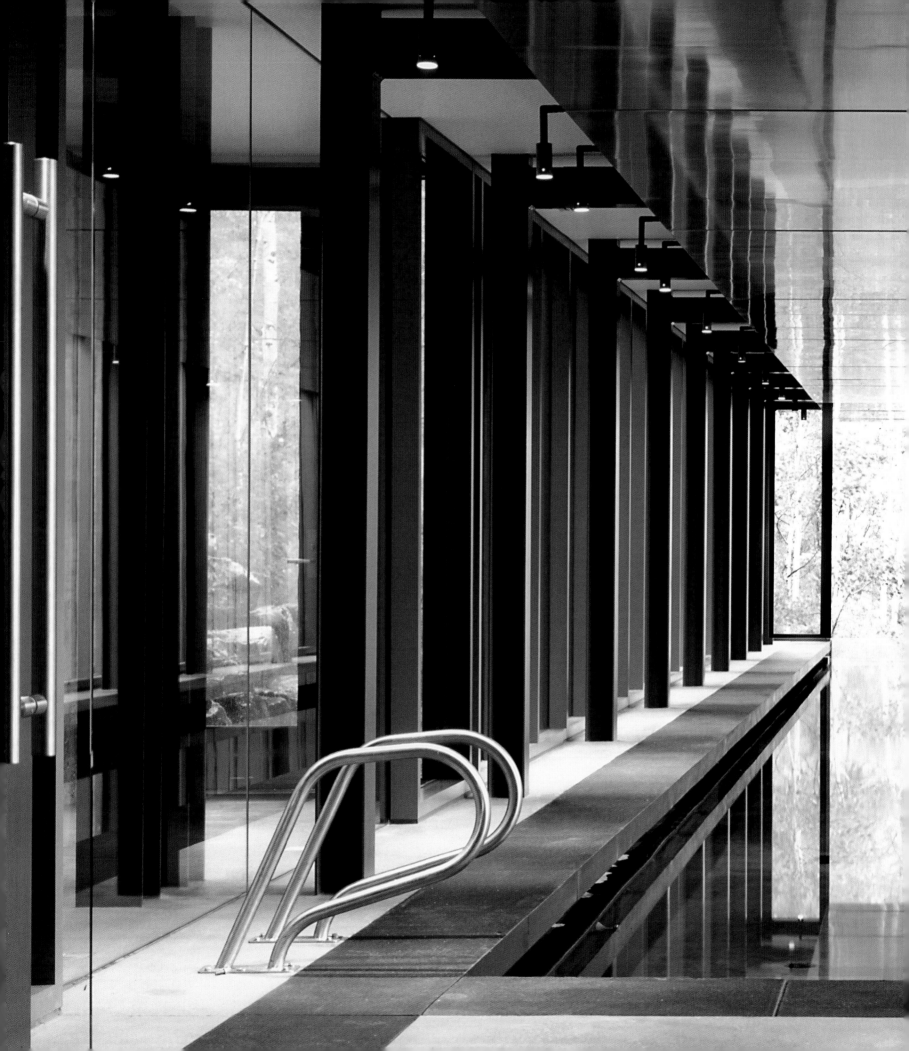

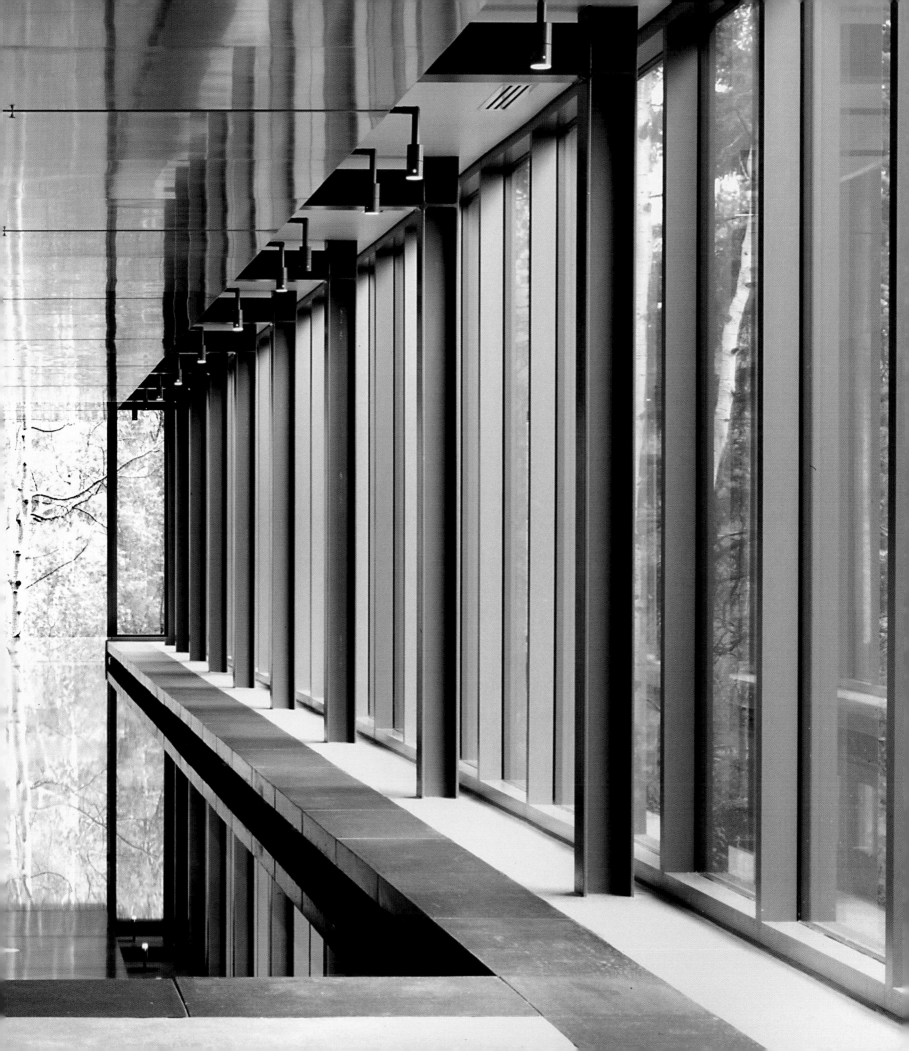

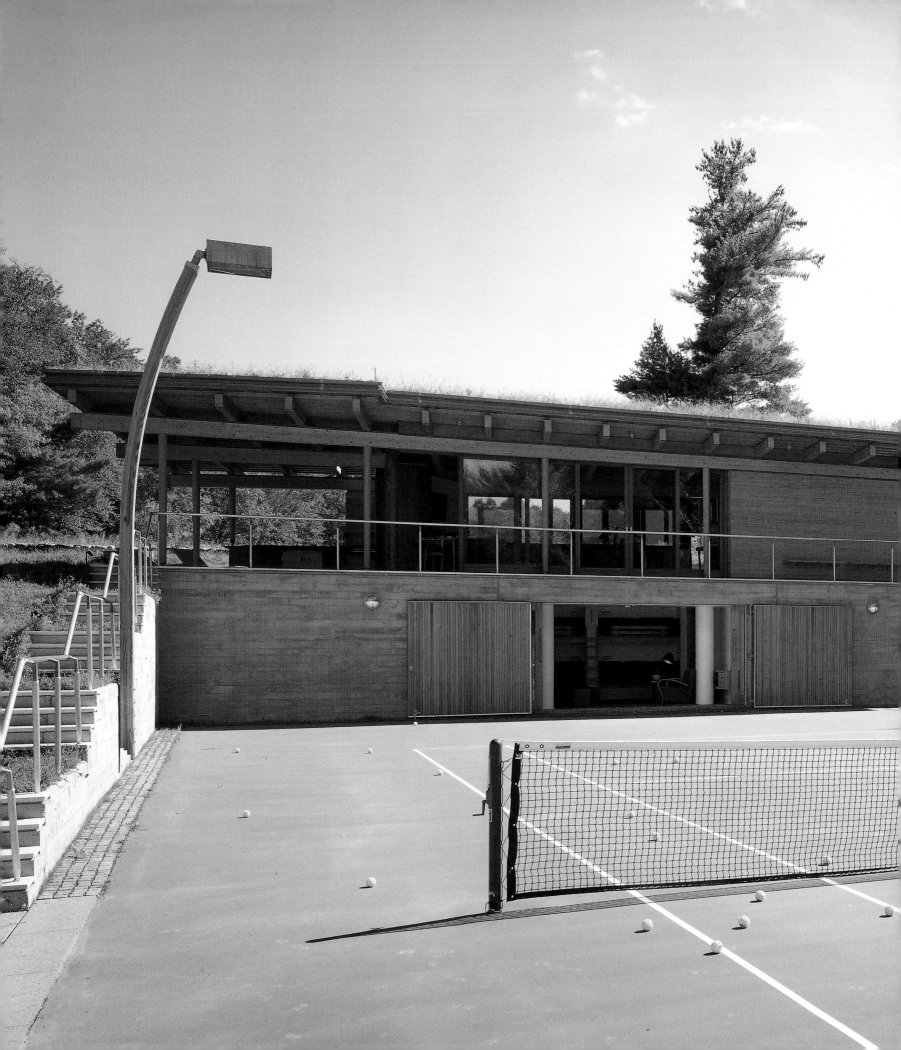

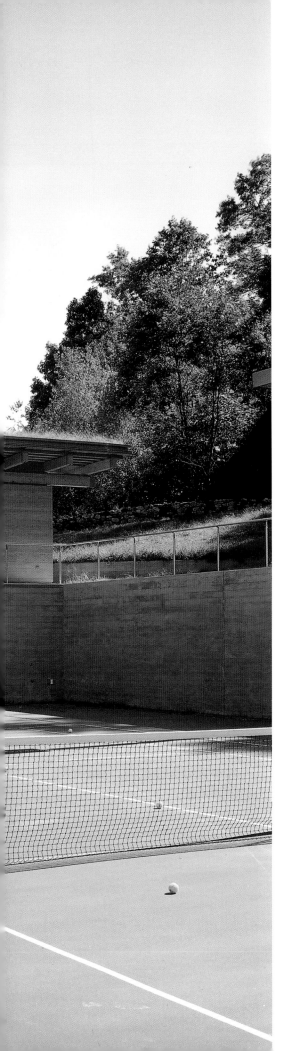

Tennis, Anyone?

THE TENNIS HOUSE

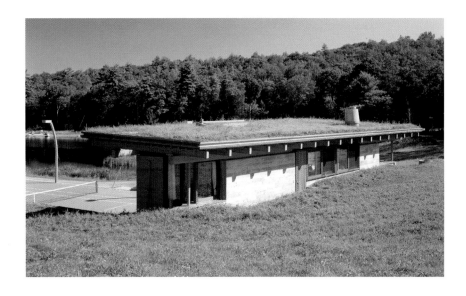

LEFT: Enthusiasm for the game of tennis prompted the owners of this Connecticut land tract to complete their tennis /guesthouse before putting the finishing touches on the main house. ABOVE: Built in an artificial valley formed by a quarry operation, the tennis court appears to have been cut into the surface of the meadow. The tennis house's green roof of wild grasses, flowering weeds, and sedum helps to visually integrate it into its surroundings and, as a practical measure, provides insulation.

IF YOU BUILD IT, WILL THEY come and play? One fitness haven designed to nurture both the healthy goals of the homeowners and the health of the new home's environment proves they will. The architects Lisa Gray and Alan Organschi were commissioned to create a home and guesthouse at a former gravel quarry in northern Connecticut. Their mission was to build structures that would not only facilitate exercise, but also heal a site ravaged by decades of excavation.

"The landscape looked like a moon crater," said Organschi of the devastated site. Today, wildflowers and meadow grass again soften the valley's outline, and the new buildings merge graciously into the revival. Although construction began on both structures at the same time, the smaller, 800-square foot tennis

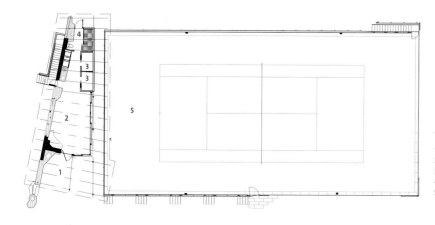

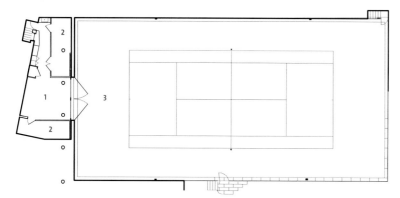

VIEWING LEVEL

1　Terrace/Overlook
2　Living Room
3　Changing Room
4　Bath
5　Tennis Court

COURT LEVEL

1　Bunk Room with Sitting Area
2　Mechanical/Storage
3　Tennis Court

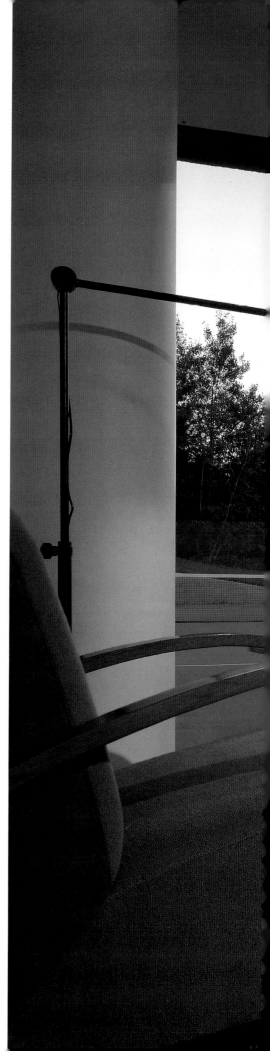

house/guest house was finished first and immediately put to good use. "The client and his children are great tennis players," said Organschi. "They use the court constantly."

The tennis house was built in the small, artificial valley formed over time by a quarry operation. It was only after the town's conservation commission called a halt to the sale of gravel from the site that the slow process of healing the land could begin. A land developer started the process by reshaping the land into a hardscrabble bowl surrounding a small spring-fed pond.

The tennis court was cut into the southwestern edge of a basin that forms the pond. Board-formed concrete retaining walls shape the enclosure on three sides of the court. The other corner of the court—exposed by the falling grade—is hemmed by a removable curtain of woven net, suspended from a tensioned cable. The tops of the concrete walls match the

RIGHT: The tennis house is also suited to spectator sport. Games in progress may be viewed from slatted wooden lawn chairs on the sunny second-story deck, from the upper level's living room, or from comfortable armchairs inside the ground-floor bunk room. In between retrieving stray balls, the bunk room is also a comfortable place to watch the sun set—over a shimmering pond and behind the blue-green wooded hills.

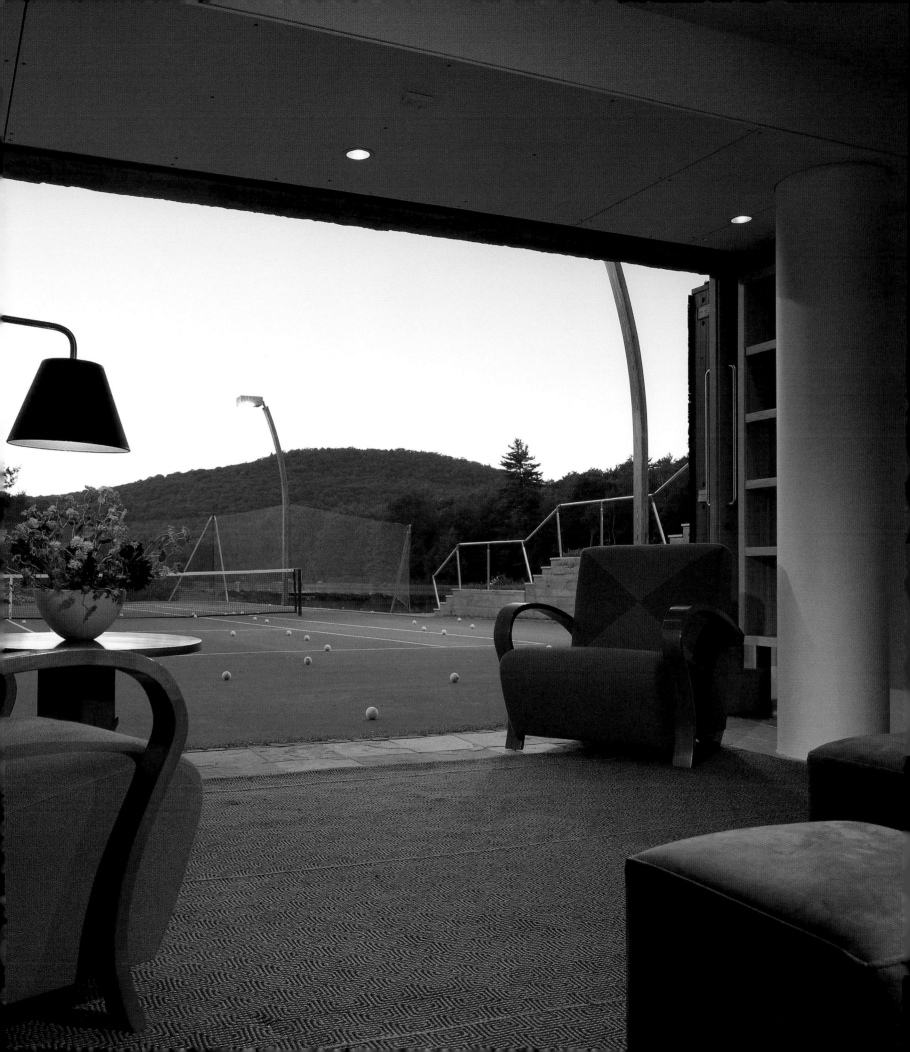

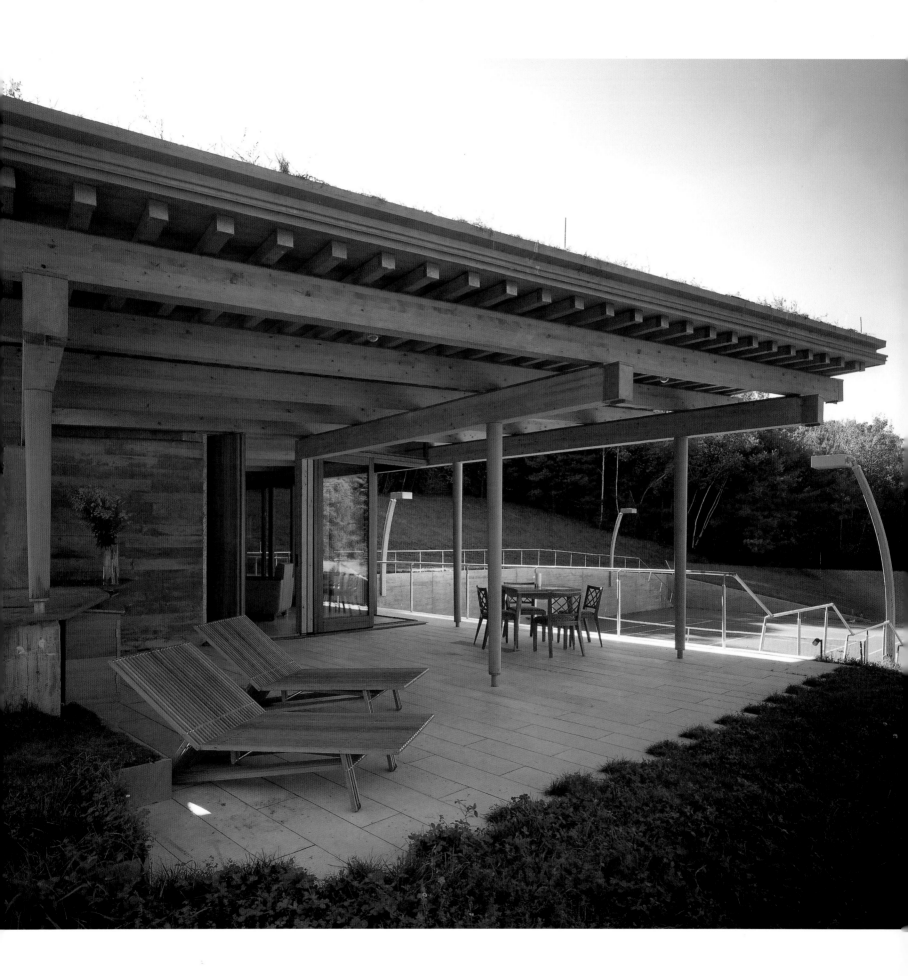

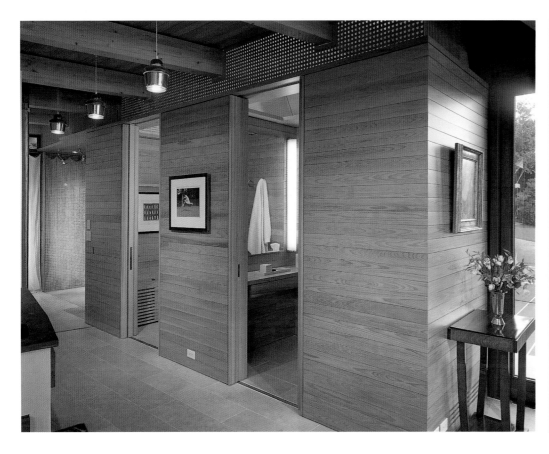
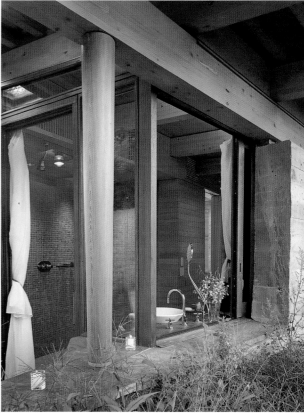

LEFT: Using old growth and recycled cypress for its window frames, walls, and doors, the tennis house makes a strong environmental statement. ABOVE, LEFT and RIGHT: Conservation easement limited interior space to a modest 600 feet and yet the house still contains two changing rooms (left), a bathroom (right), a kitchenette, a laundry for those tennis whites, a bunk room and sitting room at court level, equipment storage rooms, and a living room overlooking the court.

natural elevations of the surrounding site and rise and fall with the grade of the hillside. The court appears to have been neatly cut into the otherwise undisturbed surface of the meadow as it slopes toward the water's edge.

At the south end of the tennis court, heavy doors—sided, like all the building's doors, with boards milled from salvaged cypress timbers— swing open to a small bunk room and sitting area at court level, embedded into the hillside. Seated in the bunk room's comfortable chairs, you have only to reach out and grab a tennis ball to get in the game.

Above, the small house overlooks the court. The concrete retaining wall that forms the building's back elevation transforms along its length to create an exterior shower, a sink counter for the bathroom, a storage wall containing the kitchenette and laundry, a rear stair to the court-level spaces, an interior fire-

place and an exterior grill, and ultimately a catch basin for the roof's rainwater runoff.

The house is about a quarter of a mile away on the other side of the pond. It has six bedrooms and three levels with small barn-like wings that surround a central courtyard. The ground floor base is embedded into a steep hillside that overlooks the former gravel pit. With its large, westward-facing windows, the ground-floor level contains the exercise area, squash court, and a sauna. The exercise space overlooks a 12-by-50-foot pool that runs right up to a sliding glass wall. On the other side of the glass is an outdoor spa hot tub. The setting creates the illusion that the water goes through the glass; on warm days you can slide the glass open.

Fitness dictated the home's dimensions. When it came to pouring foundations, the squash court drove the plan of the house.

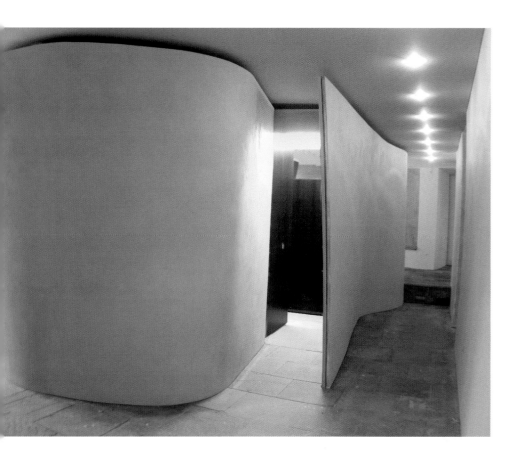

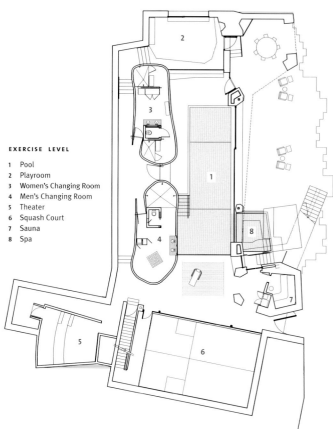

EXERCISE LEVEL

1 Pool
2 Playroom
3 Women's Changing Room
4 Men's Changing Room
5 Theater
6 Squash Court
7 Sauna
8 Spa

Excavating just the right space was important since the court had to be 21 feet wide (and at least 18-and-a-half feet high), as is designated by international squash-playing rules.

Privacy—another essential element in a workout—was also factored into the home's design. Planning ensured that it is possible to get out of the master bedroom quietly and have a full morning workout before the day starts. The fitness-focused layout makes it easier to get downstairs without waking everyone, to swim a few laps and work out on the treadmill, use the changing room as a bathroom and dressing room, then climb back up two flights of stairs, getting a further workout with each step.

The changing rooms, swimming pool, Ping-Pong, and squash areas all were sized for heavy use by a large family. Although the other rooms on the ground floor have stone-tile floors, the squash court has a sprung wooden floor. A 14-by-14-inch piece of flooring inset is used to create air space under the floorboards. This provides a flexible wood floor that's slightly soft. Before construction was even complete, the first family holiday saw round-the-clock squash tournaments in the new court. "You can provide a venue for healthy people to really play and work out all the time and they'll do it despite the fact that the house might not be completed," said Organschi.

The way the buildings sprawl out over the 200-acre woodland property might also boost the scores on a pedometer. Paths connect the buildings, while interesting trails on surrounding old farmland forests on the deeply wooded hillsides invite hiking. "The whole idea of using the land as a place for health became internalized in a great way;

ABOVE: Although the tennis house is only a quarter of a mile away, there are plenty of opportunities for fitness in the main house. Besides the swimming pool and gym area, the main house also has Ping-Pong and squash playing areas enjoyed by the whole family. Men's and women's changing rooms can be used to shower and get dressed for work.
RIGHT: The fitness-focused layout of the main house makes it easier for any member of the family to rise early, swim a few laps, and work out on the treadmill before anyone else rises.

high fit home

the ethic of trying to restore the damaged landscape became ingrained in the way we wanted the buildings to blend into the landscape," said Organschi.

The most effective blending takes place on the roofs of both houses. The roof of the home's lower floor, which extends out and stretches into a courtyard, and the guesthouse roof are both covered in grass and sod. In the three-inch soil layer on the guesthouse, sedum, wild flowers, alfalfa, and vetch grow. The whole roof system was designed to retain water, irrigating the grass.

The tennis building is heated and cooled entirely by a ground-source heat pump that uses the water of the quarry pond as a thermal mass. By avoiding the use of fossil fuels, the system, tested to be safe for wildlife, has eliminated the need for gas or oil trucks to make deliveries, their paths scarring the recovering landscape.

"All that architecture can do is be provocative," said Organschi. "Architecture can't force you to live a certain way, but good air, ventilation, lovely light, and character can make people want to use a space."

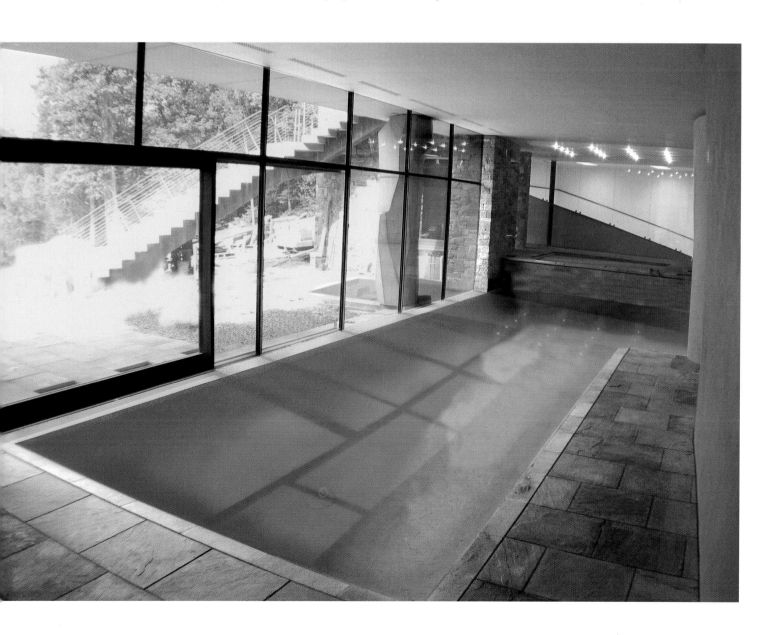

Gym with a View

THE VXO HOUSE

PEOPLE WHO LIVE IN GLASS HOUSES may not want to throw rocks, but the people who work out in the glass gym designed for the VXO house by Alison Brooks feel perfectly comfortable lifting weights.

The idea behind the VXO house in Hampstead, London was to create a new "domestic campus" of structures that integrate landscape, structural form, and site-specific art into a visual and spatial narrative. The new campus configuration has added not only a space to work out in, but a reason to walk in the garden.

The campus includes the "V" house, the "X" pavilion gymnasium/guesthouse, and the "O" port, a combination garden pavilion and carport. The extension to the original 1960s house was conceived as an opaque, timber-clad volume hovering over an open, glass-enclosed foyer space. This box is supported by one bright red "V" column and pinned back to the existing structure at the ground floor level. The house conversion entailed creating large openings in cross walls and creating a large double height gallery over the dining area. These openings connect living spaces horizontally, vertically, and to the garden, so that the house is fully illuminated with natural light.

A new foyer space, with the floor set one step lower than the existing ground floor to delineate the old and new, is the setting for three principle "events," the "V" column, a new suspended stair hung from the second

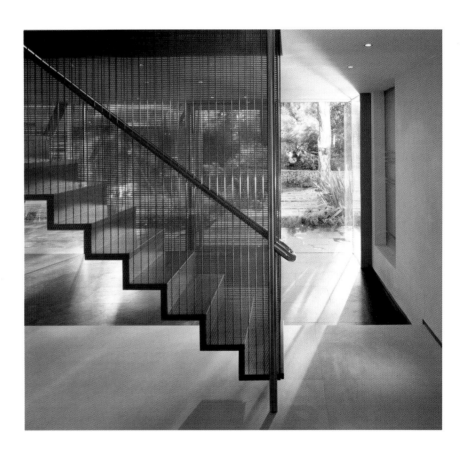

ABOVE and RIGHT: This domestic campus of structures makes no secret of the importance of exercise. Rather than a gazebo, the grounds of the VXO house contain a glass-enclosed gymnasium/guesthouse. The Hampstead, London house includes the main "V" house with its spare yet elegant interiors, the "X" pavilion garage, which faces the home's "V," and the "O" port, a combination garden pavilion and carport.

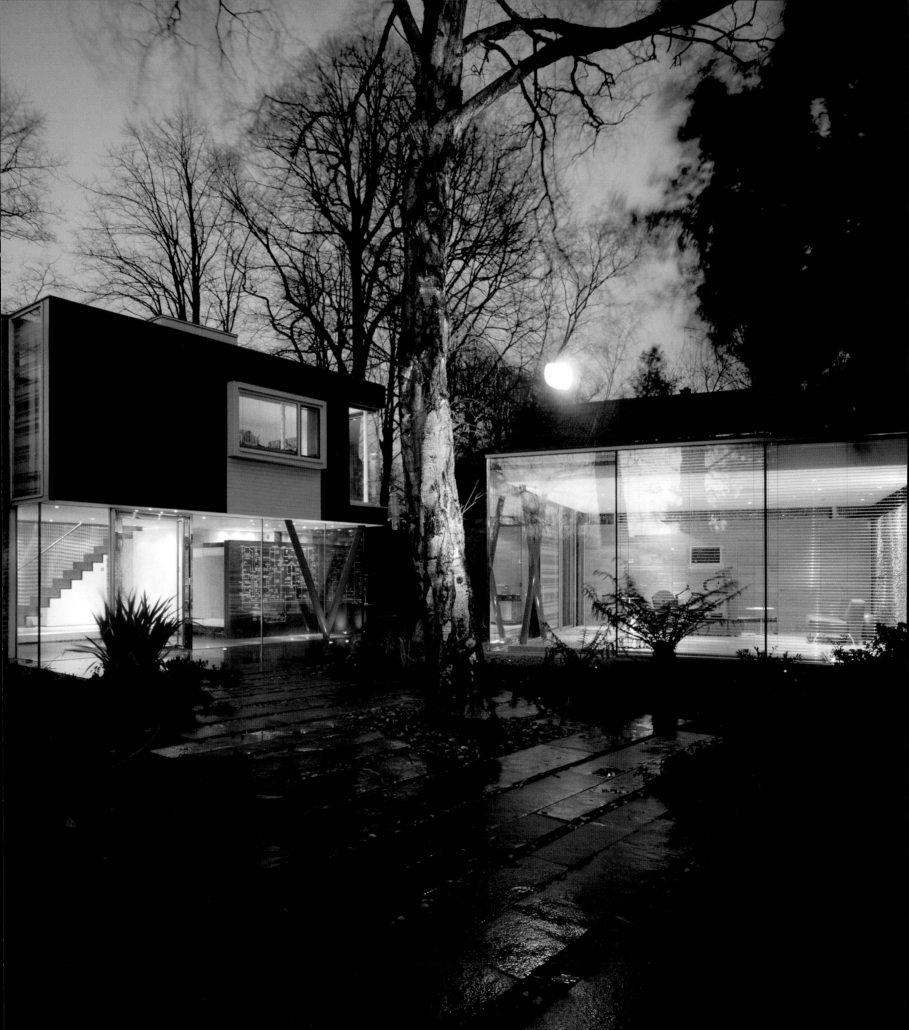

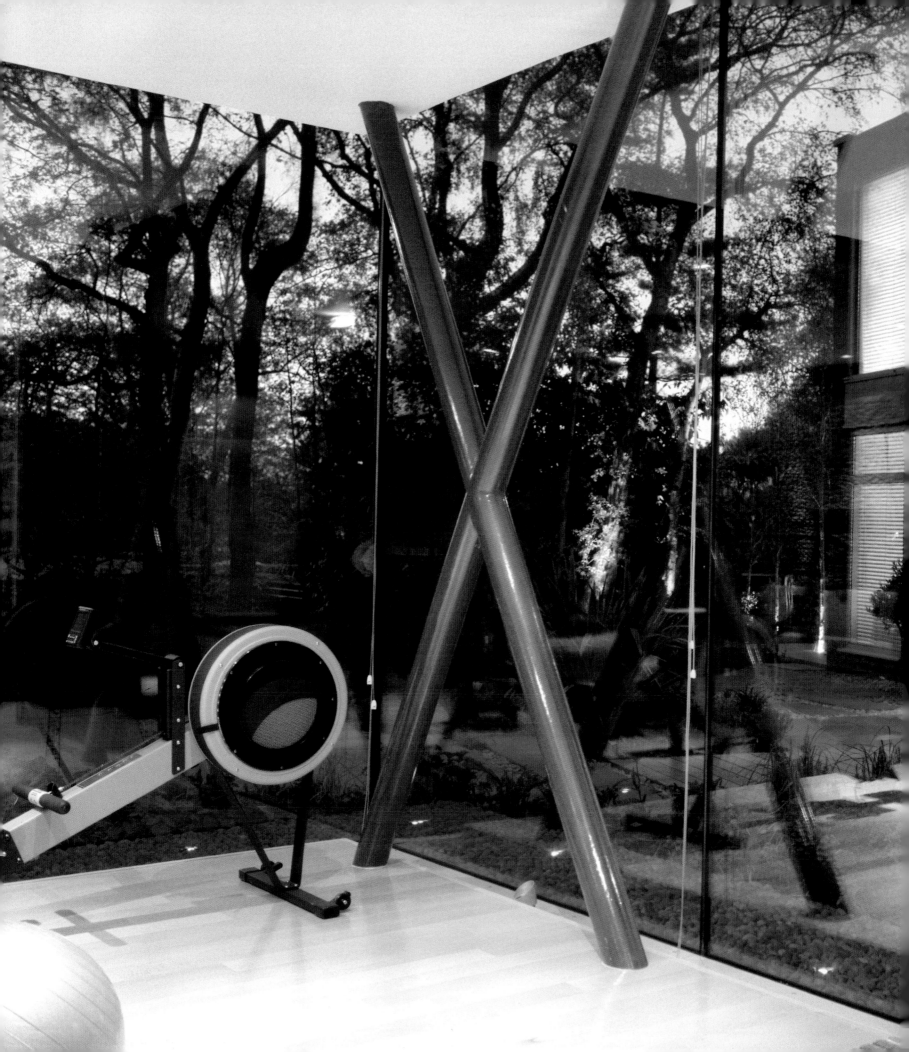

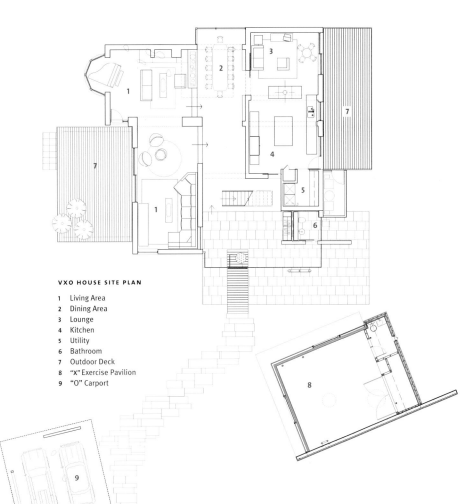

VXO HOUSE SITE PLAN

1 Living Area
2 Dining Area
3 Lounge
4 Kitchen
5 Utility
6 Bathroom
7 Outdoor Deck
8 "X" Exercise Pavilion
9 "O" Carport

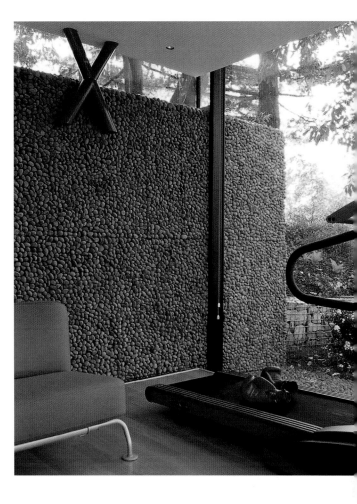

LEFT: Not only does the lean aesthetic of the former garage—now a highly visible gym—encourage fitness efforts, the walk there adds a health-inducing few steps. **RIGHT:** The home's teenagers enjoy spending time in the guesthouse/gym and having sleepovers there. It is far enough away to seem like their own space and yet close enough for parents to oversee— and if the teens happen to work out, all the better. The pebbled interior wall of the gym provides a textural contrast with the gleaming exercise equipment and the smooth glass exterior.

floor with walls of stainless-steel mesh, and a freestanding screen wall that extends from the interior to the exterior terrace.

The "X" pavilion was conceived as an assembly of landscape elements (garden roof, timber deck, pebble wall, zinc shed) superimposed, folded together, and joined with a transparent skin. Like two cupped hands superimposed, the pavilion's folded plates make the building face two directions simultaneously, toward the property entrance and the house opposite.

The building's primary enclosing element is a folded plate of in situ concrete that forms both the retaining wall and a plinth on which the pavilion sits. The second element is a folded timber plate superimposed on the plinth as a floor that folds vertically to form a

wall. This vertical timber wall screens a shower room, a cabinet, and a storage room.

The sedum roof of the pavilion is the garden—displaced to become a lawn for the second-floor bedroom opposite. This "tray of greenery" is lifted completely clear of the pavilion by two anthropomorphic structural "X"s. The green roof is punctured by two large oculi so the tree canopy can be viewed as a second arboreal roof for the pavilion.

The gymnasium's guestroom stands in the space originally reserved for a double-car garage. To add the necessary volume to the house would have blocked the landscape and cut rooms off from light and the garden.

"By creating a pavilion," said Brooks, "we were making the home larger without making the footprint bigger. It was also about the

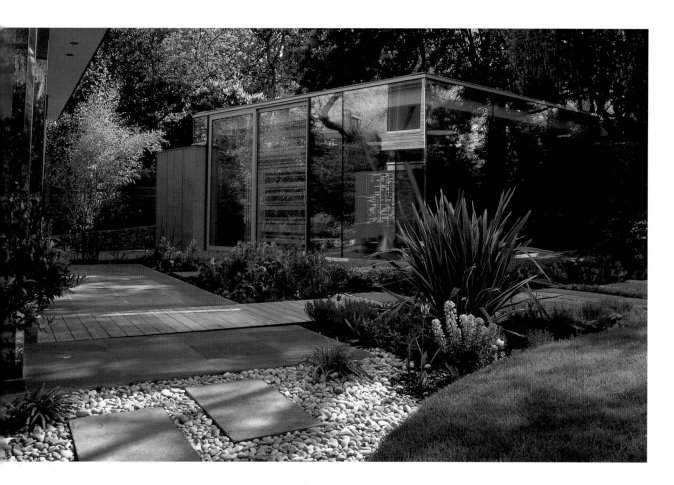

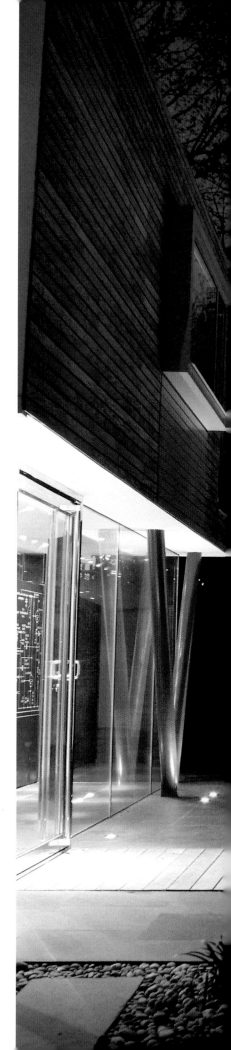

idea of pavilions and partitions in the garden, having somewhere to walk to. You have to go through the garden to get to the gym."

The gym is much appreciated by the young teenagers who live in the house and use the gym to hang out in and for sleepovers. The homeowners enjoy working out in the glass gym, because they can look out and see the gardens.

"There are no mirrors in this gym because it's more about doing something in the garden," said Brooks. You can see a corner of the gym from the street but the glass walls are so reflective that the structure disappears into its mirroring surface, becoming indistinguishable from the surrounding vegetation.

No longer hidden, workout spaces have become a proud asset to the state-of-the-art home.

ABOVE: During the day, the glass gymnasium almost seems transparent, at best some structural sculpture in the garden. RIGHT: At night, when the gym is well lit, you can see only a sliver of the interior from the street but the highly reflective nature of the glass provides privacy. The gym makes the home larger without changing the size of the footprint.

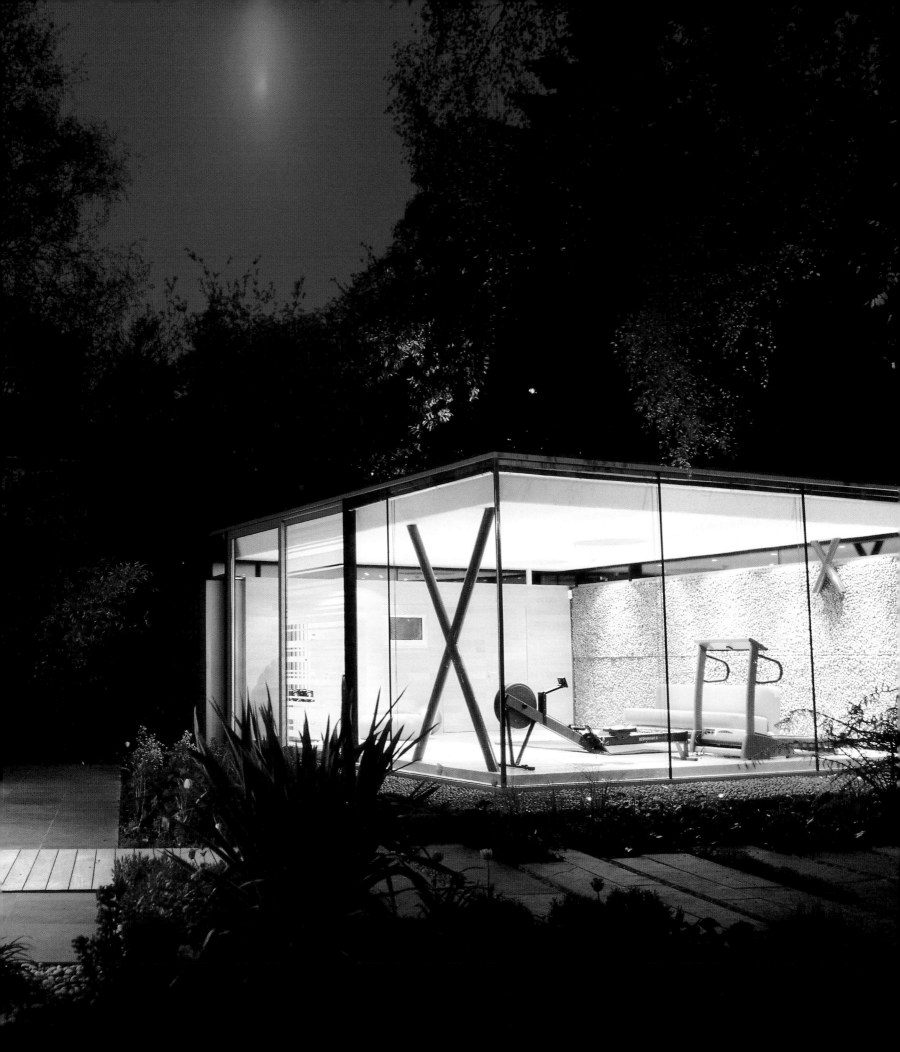

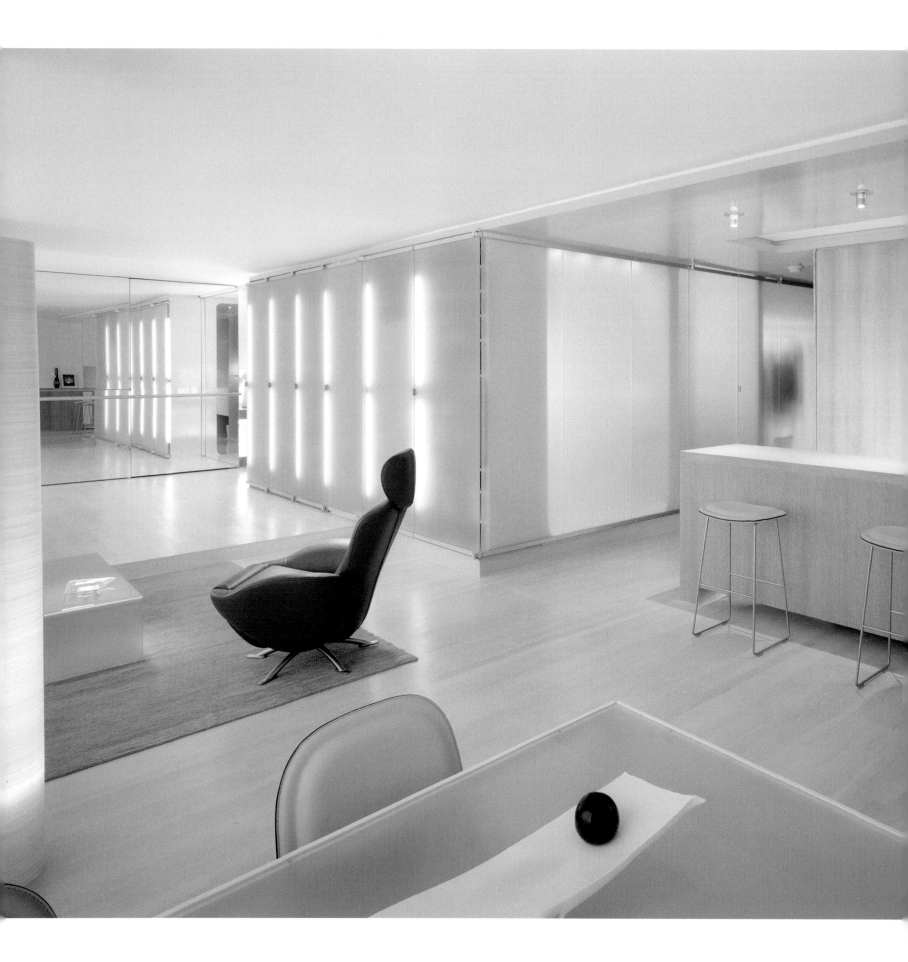

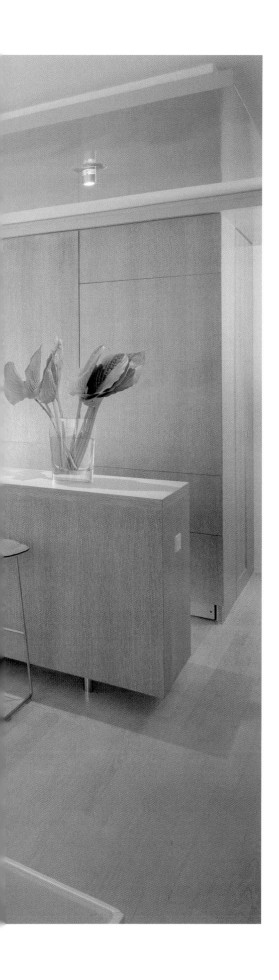

Flex Space for Dancers

THE MILLENNIUM APARTMENT

IN NEW YORK CITY, where space is always at a premium, one effective way to incorporate exercise is to create a workout room that can—at a moment's notice—be put to another use, such as accommodating overnight guests. In the Millennium Apartment, an 1,800-square-foot gut renovation, Joel Sanders took a two-bedroom uptown apartment and created a continuous, yet flexible open space, reminiscent of a downtown loft.

The first design decision Sanders made was to raze the existing walls that divided the space into a series of isolated rooms and create a pliable open plan, with space for and a resilient floor conducive to ballet practice. The room is also designed to be used as a spare bedroom for out-of-town guests and to provide storage space. "It's important to create multifunctional space and not sacrifice square footage for something you only use for a few hours a day," he said.

Every square foot of the floor area is designed to assume a variety of functions. In the ballet practice room, mirrored walls reflect each *pas de deux*, but also double as closet doors, with the ballet barre serving as a handle to open them. Within one closet is a Murphy bed that can be pulled down for additional sleeping accommodations.

When guests arrive, concealed panels unfold to convert the dance-practice area into a private guest suite. Similarly, pivoting panels

LEFT: With space at a premium in New York City, dancers have to get creative if they want to polish their *pas de deux*. In this apartment, with the feel of a loft, a dance space doubles as a guest room. The mirrored walls make the 1,800-square-foot space seem even larger and add the ambience of a loft. Sleek fittings serve to enhance the spacious feeling and not detract from it.

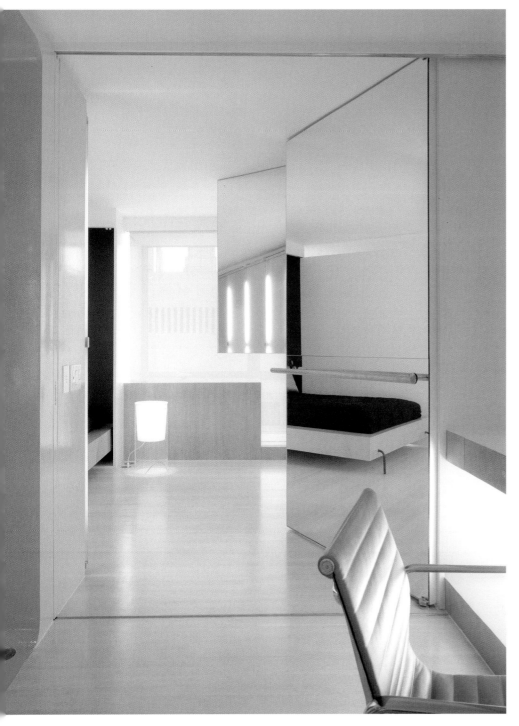

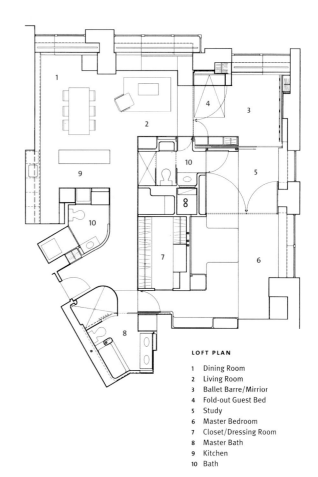

LOFT PLAN

1   Dining Room
2   Living Room
3   Ballet Barre/Mirror
4   Fold-out Guest Bed
5   Study
6   Master Bedroom
7   Closet/Dressing Room
8   Master Bath
9   Kitchen
10 Bath

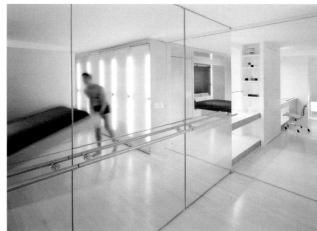

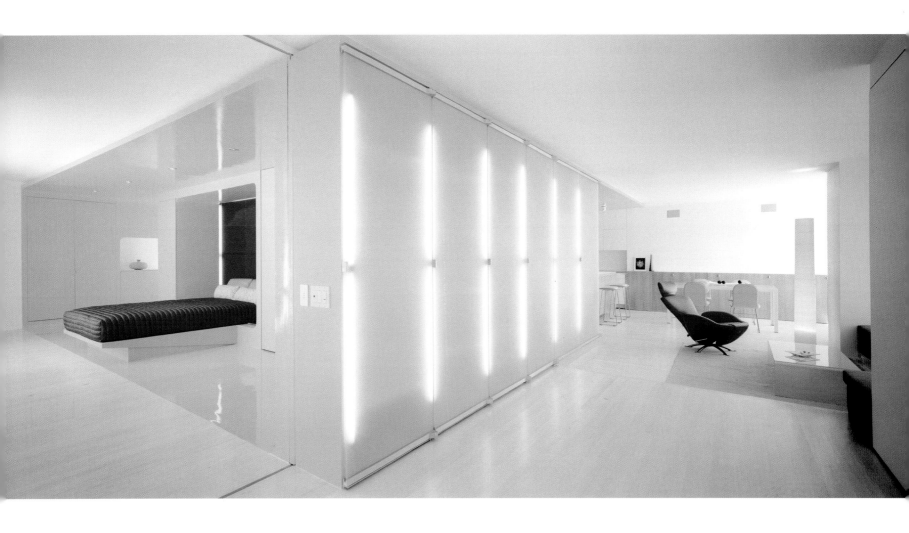

FAR LEFT: A Murphy bed pulls out from the closet to create an instant guest room. LEFT: The handles on the door serve to open storage space and access. ABOVE: The mirrored dance room is next to the living room. Being surrounded by mirrors may serve as a further incentive to get in shape.

allow the spacious bedroom to be subdivided into a private study or second guestroom.

The apartment's lean, almost seamless, luminous look was inspired by a Japanese teahouse. Its color palette of celadon green and Chinese red reinforces that influence.

The entry, living and dining area, dance-practice space, study, master bedroom, and bath form a chain of overlapping spaces that flow around a centerpiece of the project—a central service core that contains plumbing (guest bath) and storage (master closet, home entertainment, bookshelves, and appliances).

Although the opaque service unit shields contents from view, the apartment's core selectively reveals rather than conceals. Like a lantern, the translucent glass core provides the apartment's principal light source. Silhouettes of backlit bodies and household objects are veiled behind this glowing container.

Body Building for Bachelors

THE BACHELOR HOUSE

JOEL SANDERS, AN ARCHITECT committed to exploring the role architecture plays in shaping culture, has created spaces that acknowledge the importance of achieving the ideal human shape. One is a house designed for a bachelor's private workout.

Not all suburban homes are built for families. If the traditional house presupposes the nuclear family, Sanders's Bachelor House, located in a suburban Minneapolis neighborhood, reconfigures a typical developer home according to the lifestyle of the contemporary bachelor—with ample room for working out and plenty of privacy. The design, literally built on the foundations of a 1950s Rambler, reconfigures the interior in response to the bachelor's competing desires for a better view and privacy from the neighbors.

Sanders, author of *Stud: Architectures of Masculinity*, which explores concepts behind the traditional "bachelor pad," designed his bachelor home in 1998. "Suburban homes are designed for the nuclear family, but now there are all kinds of families," he said.

In the one-story, late-1950s-style house, it was not possible to build up. So a subterranean exercise space and space for a pool was created, with the suburban exterior masking the underground lair. Part of a 1999 Museum of Modern Art exhibit titled "Private Homes," the as-yet-unbuilt house features a visually deceptive AstroTurf fence.

The fence raises the level of the horizon to block out views of neighboring houses, before folding horizontally to define the soft ground covering of the backyard, where the bachelor can work out or lounge by the pool. From the subterranean floor, if you look out the window, all you see is green lawn and sky.

For Sanders, there's a direct link between personal identity, the way people exercise and clothe their bodies, and the way they build and decorate their homes. "We layer on

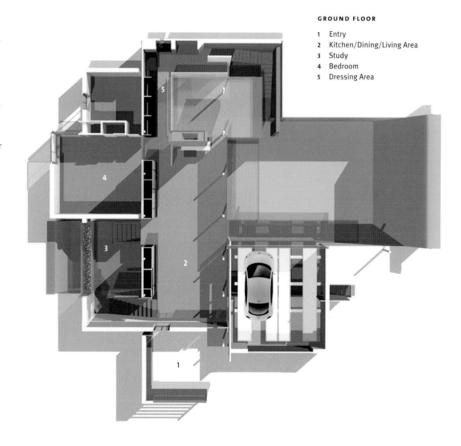

GROUND FLOOR

1 Entry
2 Kitchen/Dining/Living Area
3 Study
4 Bedroom
5 Dressing Area

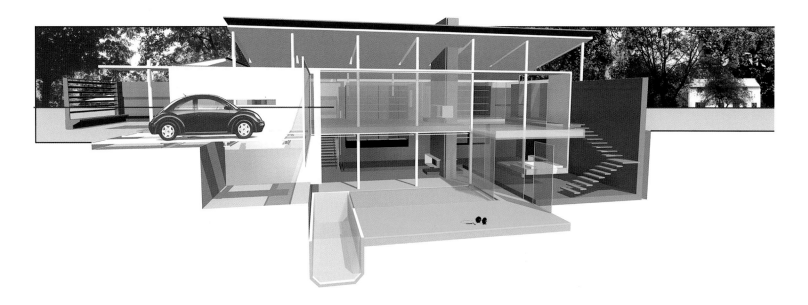

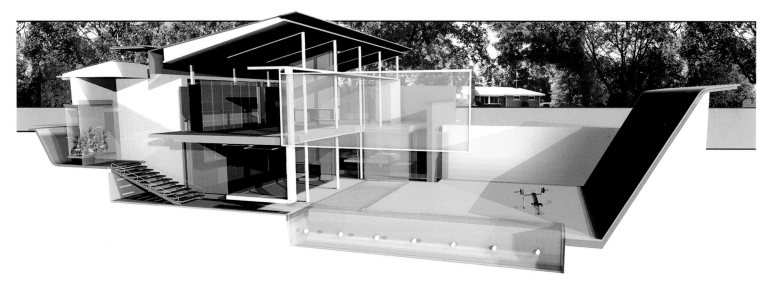

LEFT and ABOVE: Subterranean exercise space and a place for a pool are essential in the bachelor pad/suburban house designed by architect Joel Sanders. Privacy may be a priority when working out, says Sanders, so burrowing into the ground to create an enclosed oasis of fitness may be just what it takes to make exercise a daily reality.

clothing and surfaces, such as carpeting, wood, paneling, and appliances, and they create the identity of who we are."

The downstairs bachelor's bedroom contains a platform bed and windows with semi-mirrored, semi-reflective glass so the homeowner can look outside, but no one can see in. At the same time the bachelor can see himself in the mirrored walls, which contain pegs for hanging clothes.

The home features an overlapping sequence of spaces for work and leisure, zones where the bachelor can exercise his mind and body protected from the curiosity of strangers.

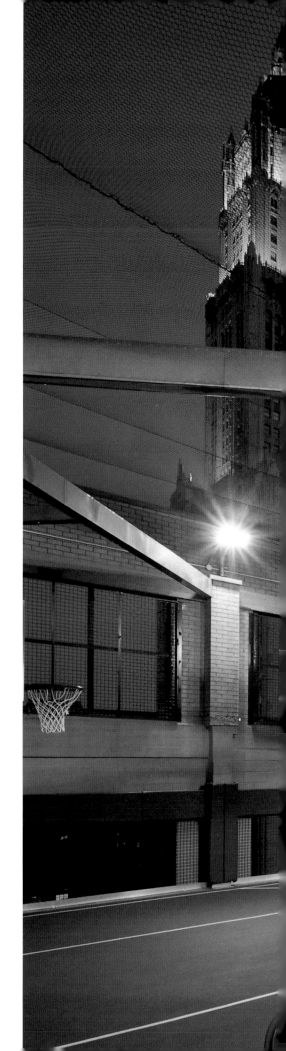

Basketball in the Sky

THE MURRAY STREET SKY COURT

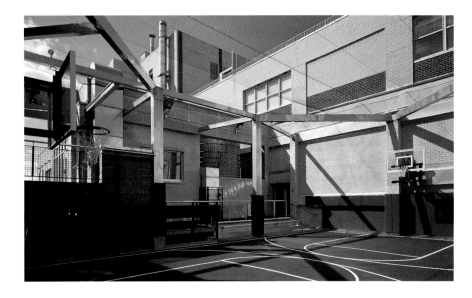

IT STARTED OUT almost as a joke during the discussion of a high-end residential building project in New York City, but the Sky Court designed by Resolution: 4 Architecture now takes the pursuit of fitness to new heights.

The architects Joseph Tanney and Robert Luntz were talking about the project with the building's developer when he jokingly asked, "Where's my basketball court?" So, they built him one—20 stories up.

The Murray Street building already has a 40,000-square-foot health club and spa, but the Sky Court adds another aspect of fitness—the communal feeling that you can only get by shooting a few hoops with the guys in the neighborhood. With seven hundred loft-size apartments, this building is a neighborhood unto itself.

ABOVE and RIGHT: With New York City real estate at a premium, sometimes the best place to incorporate a desirable feature may be up on the roof. In this Manhattan building, it's possible to shoot hoops among the stars and the glittering skyline. The court is surrounded with two-story walls to prevent balls from becoming dangerous projectiles falling to the city streets below. In addition, to keep the echo of dribbling balls from reverberating, the architects floated a new concrete slab on springs under the court's floor.

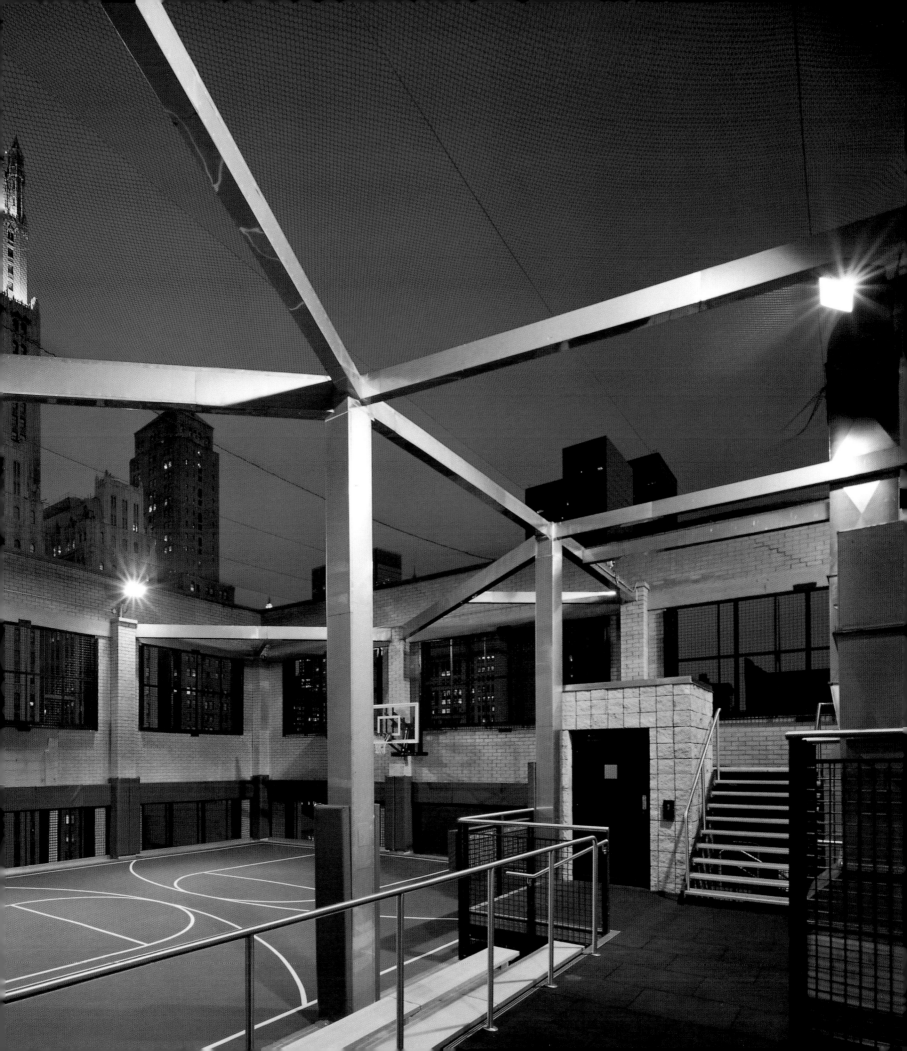

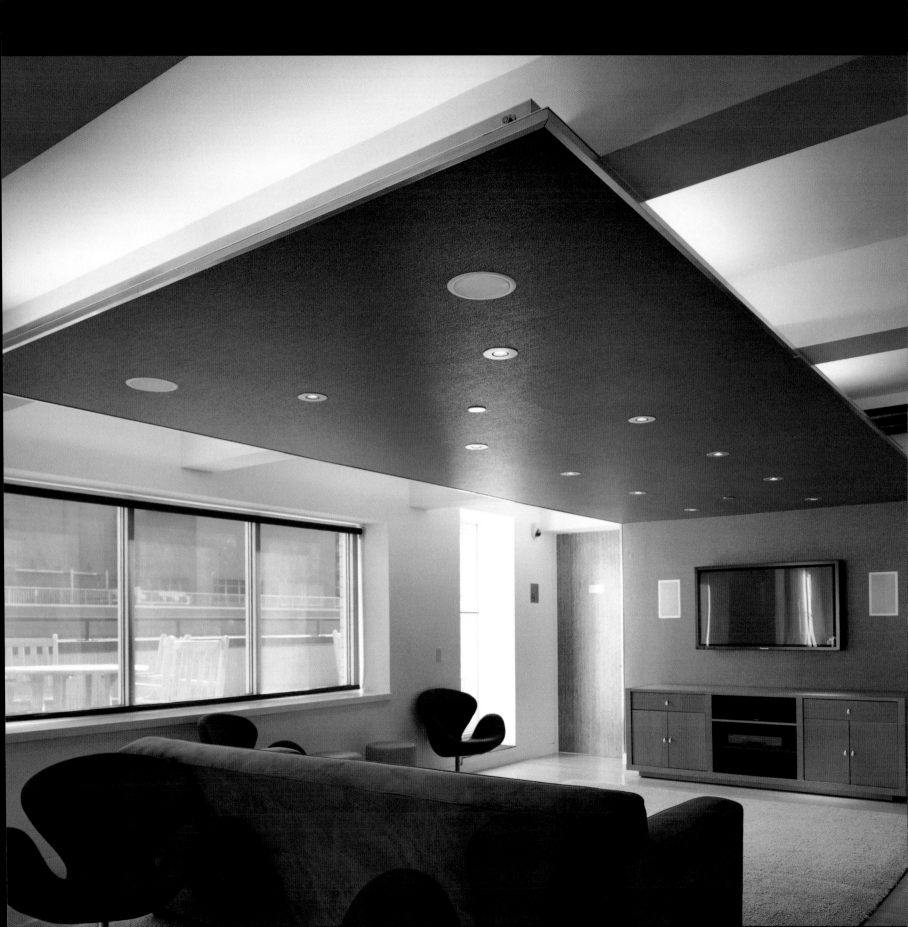

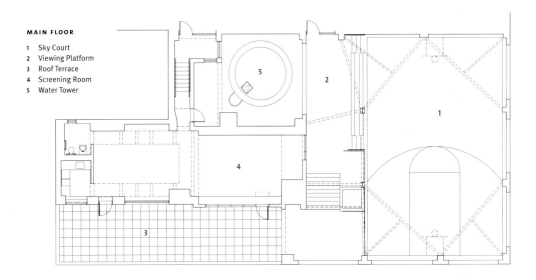

MAIN FLOOR

1 Sky Court
2 Viewing Platform
3 Roof Terrace
4 Screening Room
5 Water Tower

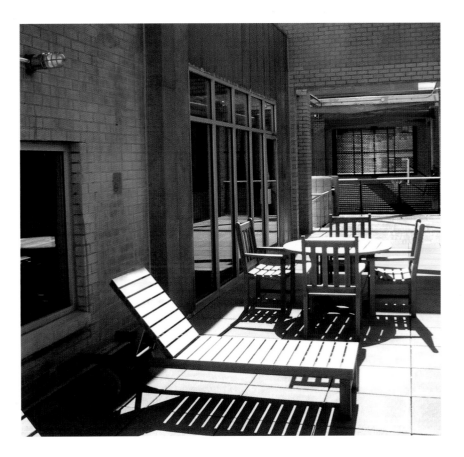

To cover the former mechanical spaces of the building's roof, the designers fashioned a complex of indoor and outdoor rooms: inside, a media room and a "playroom" with pool tables, and outside the court. All the buildings on this layer were designed to encourage a sense of community among the young professionals who live in the building—they provide a place to meet, mingle, and score a few baskets.

The rooftop buildings are huddled and layered around the existing, enclosed water tower. The remaining mechanical systems have been relocated to fit neatly under an exterior catwalk to the court. Tenants can watch games in progress from the inner rooms or from the outside bleachers—and if there's no game, they can watch the sun set through the hoop with a backdrop of the world's most famous skyline.

The 34-by-53-foot court is smaller than standard basketball-court size and was built to fit the space. To create the court, the architects had to float a new concrete slab literally on springs, so that the games' noise would not vibrate into the apartments below. To keep players from falling off the roof and to keep basketballs from becoming UFO sightings, the architects fenced in the perimeter openings with two-story windowed walls of anodized aluminum. It's the same type of aluminum used in New York City subway girders.

Why create a basketball court and not a tennis court on this rooftop? "Basketball is more of an urban thing," said Tanney.

Opening the Door

THE SINNOTT RESIDENCE

FOR THOSE WHO WANT TO shape up in this Los Angeles home, getting their feet wet is as easy as opening the living room doors. Once the doors are open, you can step directly into the blue, welcoming waters of a pool, because the angled steps culminate at the door's threshold.

"The pool is very much part of the house, part of the lifestyle," said Trevor Abramson of Abramson Teiger Architects. "Then to connect it even further, you want to be able to see the water when sitting inside."

The blue water of the pool entices residents and visitors alike, as does a spout that juts at an angle from the house to recycle the pool's water. Both the pool and the spout are visible and/or audible from several places inside the house, so they are not easily taken for granted.

Because California's friendly climate means doors can be open almost year round, many of Abramson Teiger's houses have a similarly strong indoor-outdoor interaction. Wherever you are in this house, you can see through to an adjoining space. Expansive doors and/or windows help dissolve the visual barriers between inside and outside.

Just as part of the living room juts into the pool, luring you to exercise, a gym off the master bedroom is cantilevered in space above the living room. A row of small, recessed windows and one large window in the gym

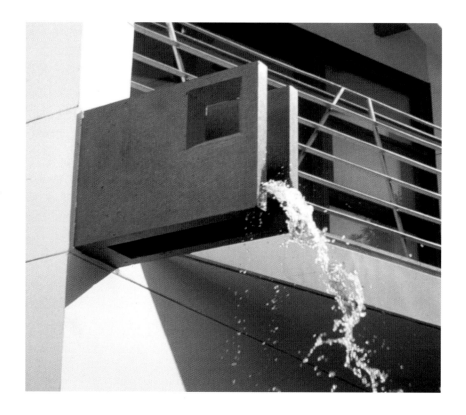

ABOVE: The weather in sunny southern California makes it easier to exercise outdoors— and so does the architecture. The water from the pool is recycled through a cleverly designed spout. From various points throughout the house, the pool or its spout is visible or audible. RIGHT: In this home, the pool is such an essential part of daily life that it is part of the augmented foundation. There is no excuse for being a couch potato when you can roll off the couch into the pool.

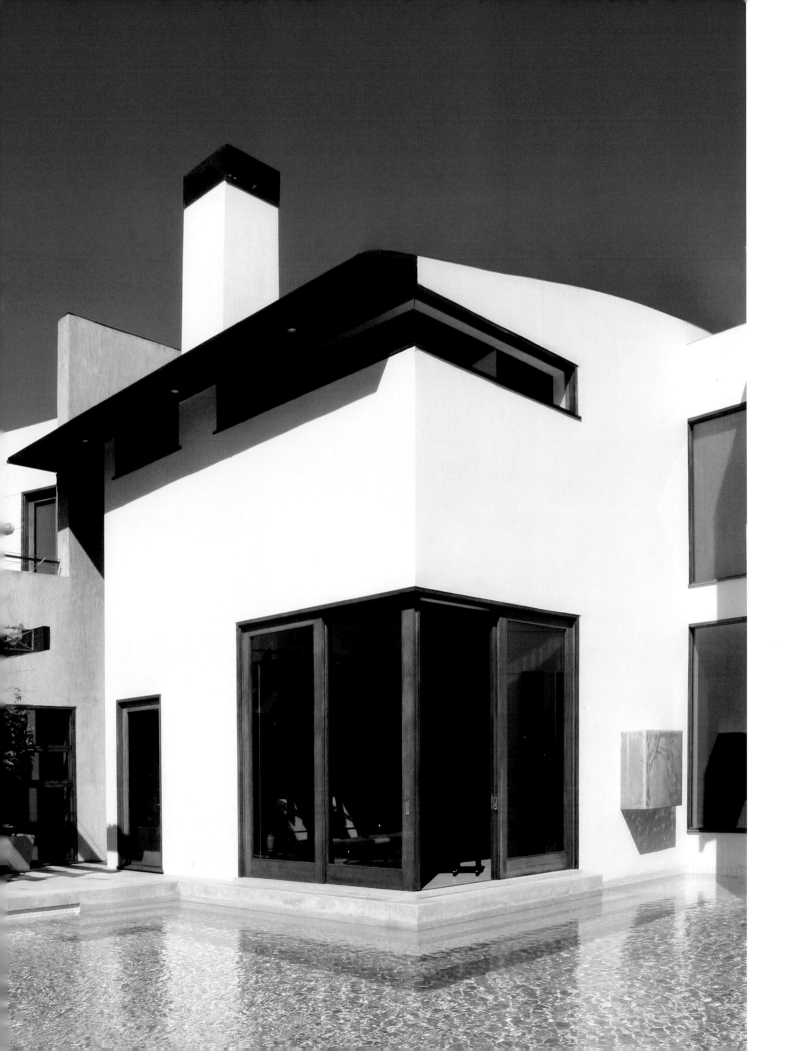

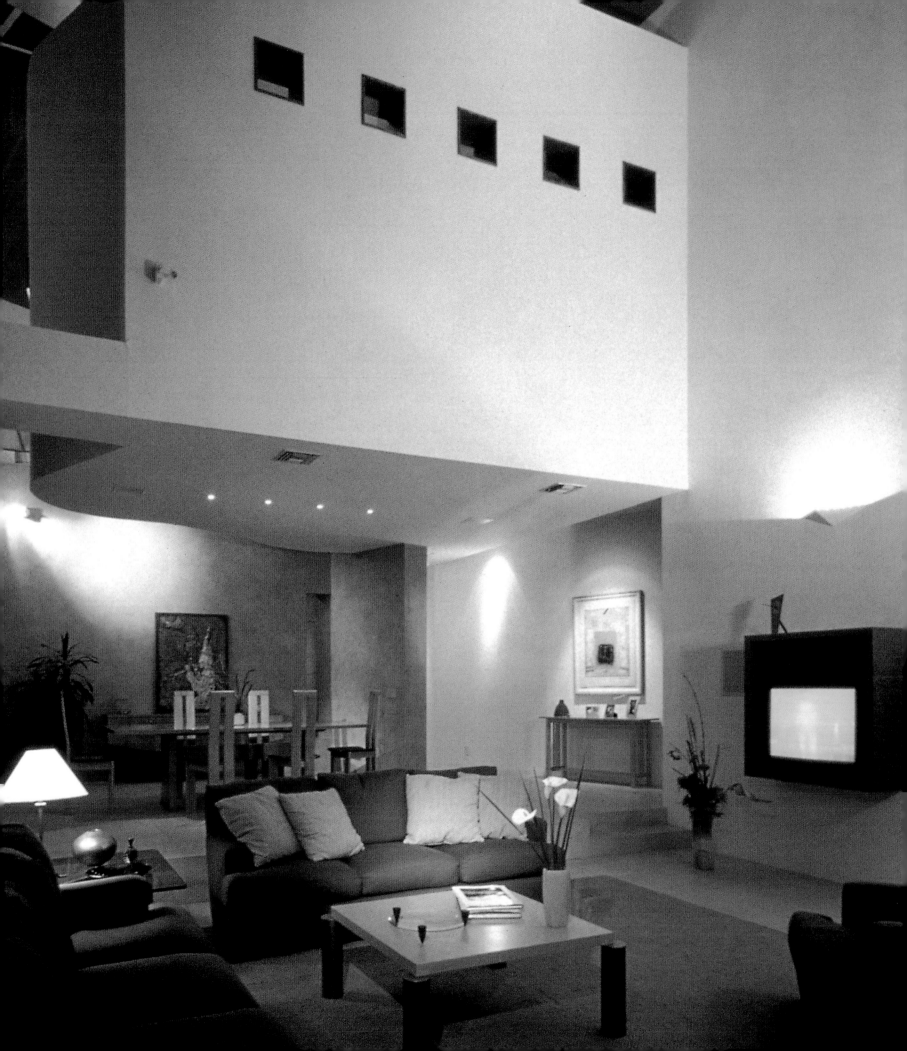

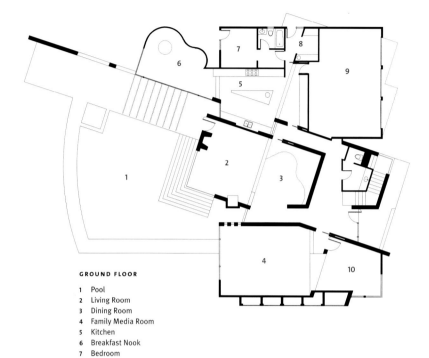

GROUND FLOOR

1 Pool
2 Living Room
3 Dining Room
4 Family Media Room
5 Kitchen
6 Breakfast Nook
7 Bedroom
8 Laundry
9 Garage
10 Study

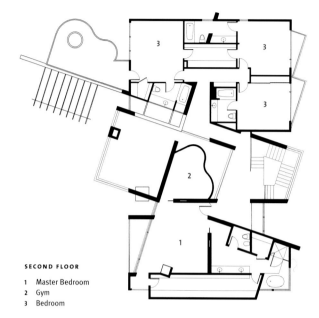

SECOND FLOOR

1 Master Bedroom
2 Gym
3 Bedroom

LEFT: The second floor in this home contains four bedrooms and a gym that remains visually connected with the first story. The porthole windows in the far wall were incorporated to afford the gym views of azure sky and blue pool water, as well as the living room. There's also a portal that looks down into the dining room, incorporating fitness into daily family life.

wall admit light and afford beautiful views during workouts.

"Although gym equipment has gotten nicer to look at and smaller, as the technology has improved, I didn't want to be looking up from the living room and see the gym, but while in the gym I wanted to be able to see garden and sky," said Abramson. The gym's windows are strategically placed above the doors that open to the pool, so trees are visible—and, of course, you can look out and see the living and dining area below.

"I've done many gyms and one of the realities of a gym is that people watch TV while exercising, which can be boring and repetitive. I think a great view invigorates the spirit," said Abramson. "It makes you feel healthy to look out and see blue sky and green leaves."

The house is all about angles and cantilevered shapes, which gives it a certain energy and a sense of movement. The central part of the house was cantilevered at a 19-degree angle, so that it opens onto a grove of trees and away from the neighbors.

The roof is slanted. Windows with no structural posts in the corner help angle the roof above. Within the building are cantilevered balconies; triangular skylights; angled step risers; glazed, angular walkways; and a trapezoidal shower/bathtub. The living room is cantilevered to meet the pool. The gym seems to float above the living room at an angle.

The suspended gym doesn't touch the sides completely or touch the roof. To provide structural support and to compensate for the added weight of gym equipment, the

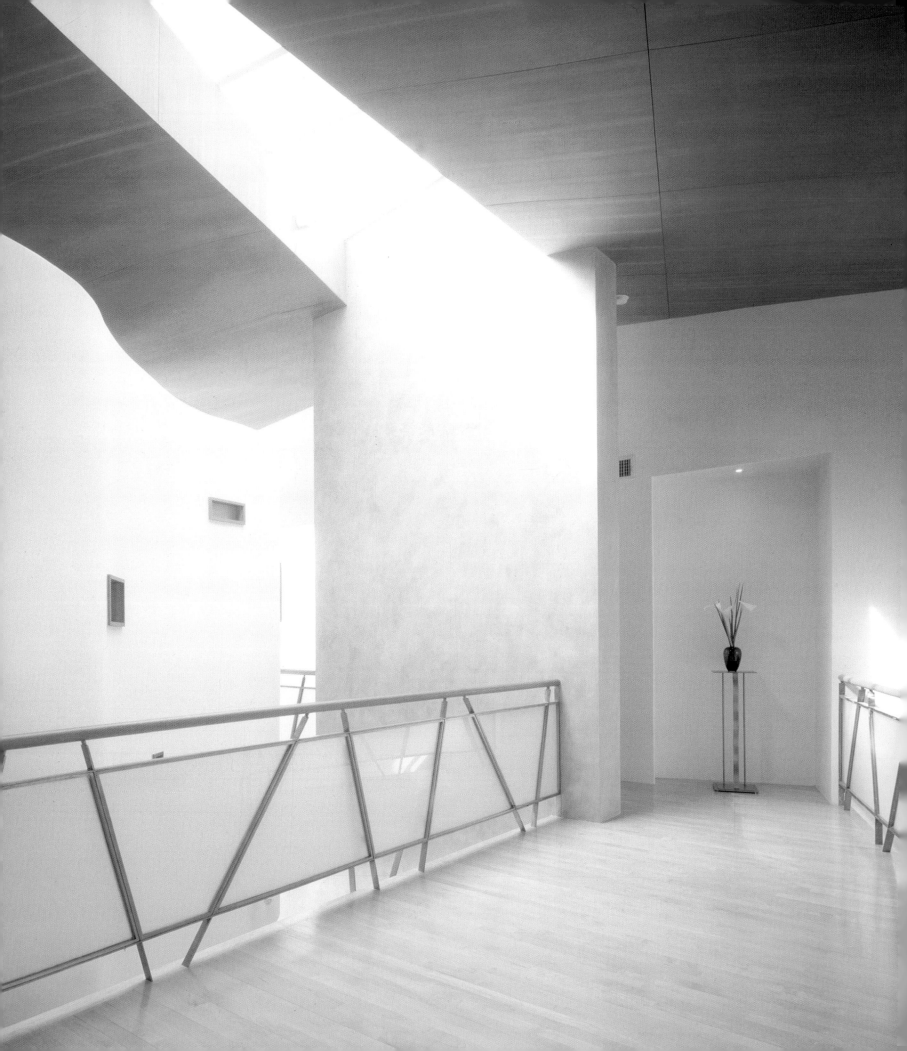

room has structural feet of steel. The steel in the floor is covered with concrete and thicker-than-normal plywood for resilience. Despite the solid construction underneath, cantilevered elements make it appear to float in space. It seems to defy gravity, which is fitting because it's all about battling the effects of gravity.

Bringing the pool up to the house also involved special structural considerations, such as augmenting the foundation to increase the support. "The structure of a pool is not designed to hold up a house. Walls of a pool that are walls of a house have to be specially designed to access both uses," said Abramson.

Most of the homes being designed by this firm typically have a gym element, a dedicated space, whether it's a room or part of a room, clearly defined as a workout space. With equipment becoming more compact and user friendly, exercise is taking a more prominent position in the house and design elements mirror this esthetic.

"Modern architecture lends itself more to the feeling of youthfulness and energy because it is light, clean, and fresh," said Abramson. "Those are all the things you are looking for in a healthier lifestyle."

LEFT: Cantilevered shapes give this "angular sensation" of a home an energetic sense of movement. ABOVE RIGHT: The view of the dining room from the gym is similar to the way a family room allows the person cooking and cleaning to interact with the family. BELOW RIGHT: The sleek modern design of the latest home equipment makes it easier to incorporate gyms into the home.

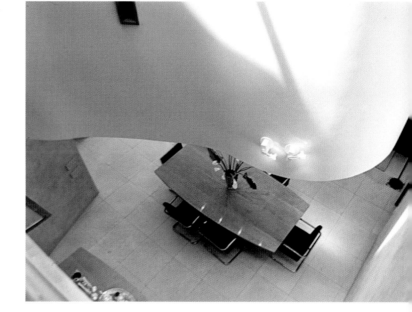

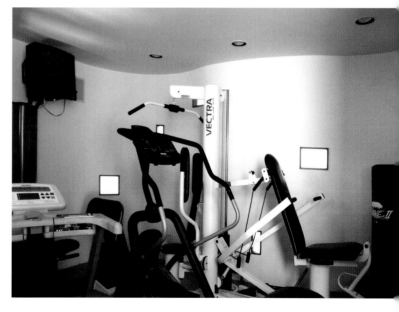

A Camp in Connecticut

THE ADIRONDACK CAMP HOUSE

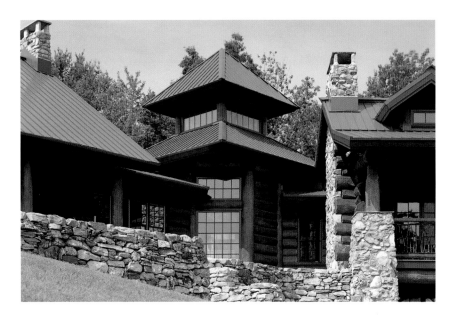

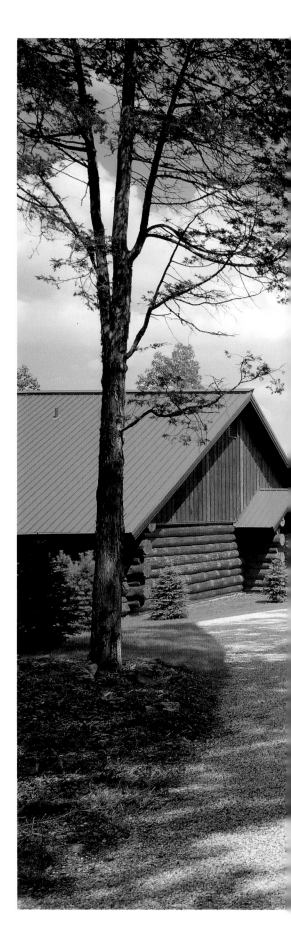

THE OWNERS OF THIS RURAL northern Connecticut site wanted a home that captured the spirit of the Great Camps of the Adirondacks—a style of resort architecture favored by wealthy industrialists and financiers between the Civil War and the Great Depression. These rustic yet well-appointed timber and stone structures, ranging from simple cabins to multi-winged Victorians, served as vacation homes for well-heeled sportsmen and women.

This camp-style home, designed by John Martin of John Martin Associates Architects, does more than evoke a bygone era. Its sprawling layout encourages its inhabitants to walk more. After studying the essential elements of the Great Camps, Martin updated them and improved the concept.

ABOVE and RIGHT: This ruggedly beautiful Adirondack-style home incorporates all the advantages of these classic vacation homes—the motivation to explore and a chance to commune with nature.

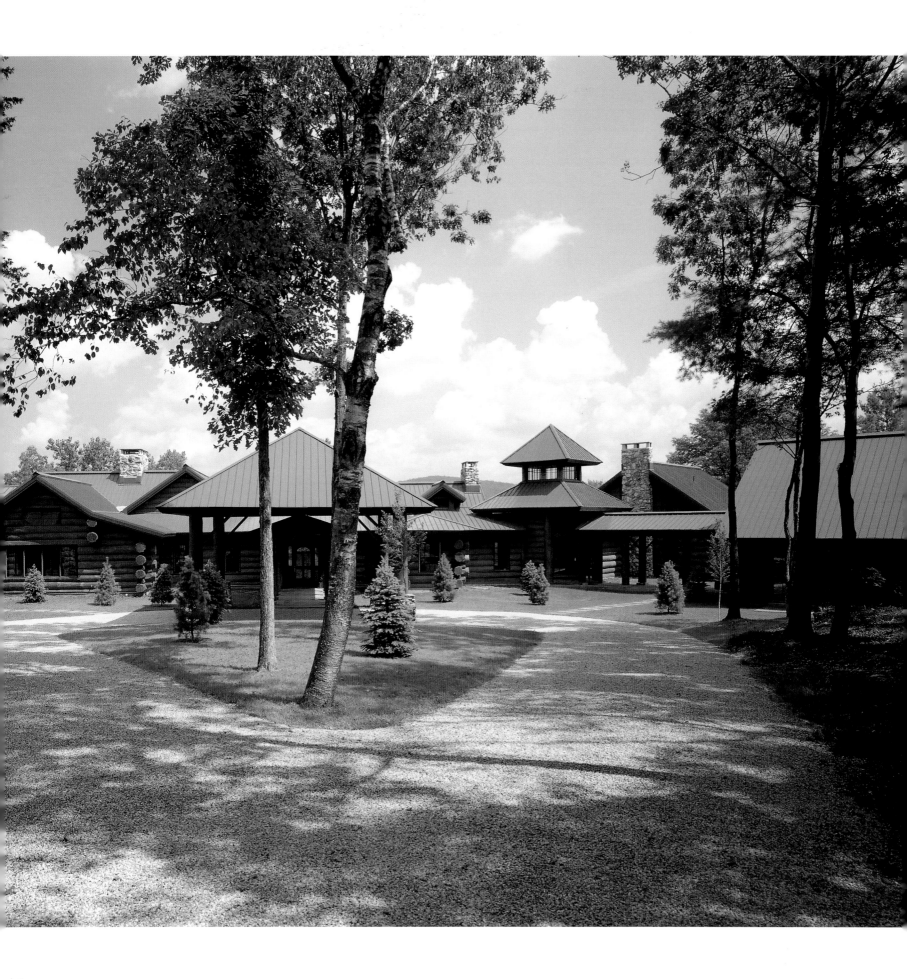

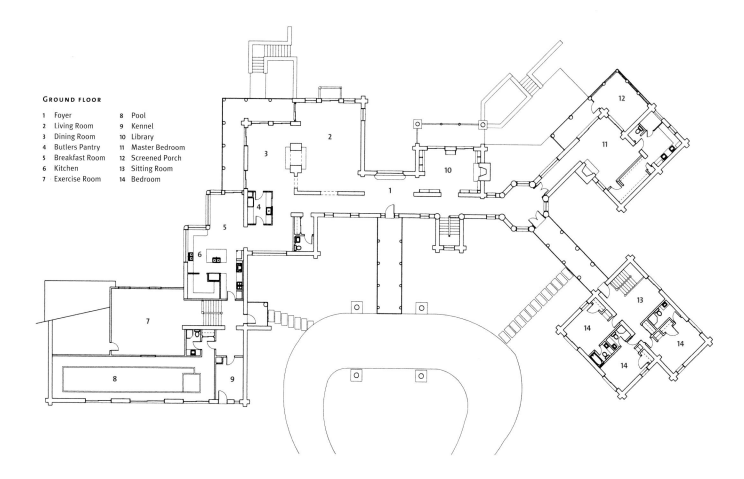

To fit neatly into and make the most of the stunning views of the surrounding mountains, Martin built a series of functional living components. He divided the house into multiple buildings or "camps" for such daily functions as sleeping, cooking, dining, or exercising. The components not only create little islands of privacy but make it easier for the house to follow the land's natural contours.

Historically, these camps comprised several buildings. You had to walk from one building to another, said Martin. Considering the area's climate extremes, he connected the cabins with enclosed walkways and, in some cases, underground tunnels.

In the Great Camp tradition, he used building materials that are or could be indigenous. Contributing to the rustic feel of the house are 18-to-24-foot lengths of northern white pine, fully scribed and handcrafted to fit into adjoining logs. All the stone was found on the site, except for the cut granite. A green standing-seam roof blends in with the surrounding foliage. Inside, each major room achieves its cozy encampment aura with a stone fireplace and wooden walls and ceilings.

"One thing the owners really appreciate are all the interesting places and views this layout creates," said Martin. "When people visit they like to walk around trying to find new things."

Camping out might not be quite so exhilarating without some form of communal exercise. Besides the exercise derived

RIGHT: Because it's really a well-thought-out spider web of buildings, connected by walkways, this home has none of the disadvantages— such getting wet or muddy— encountered when traveling between different sections of the original camps.

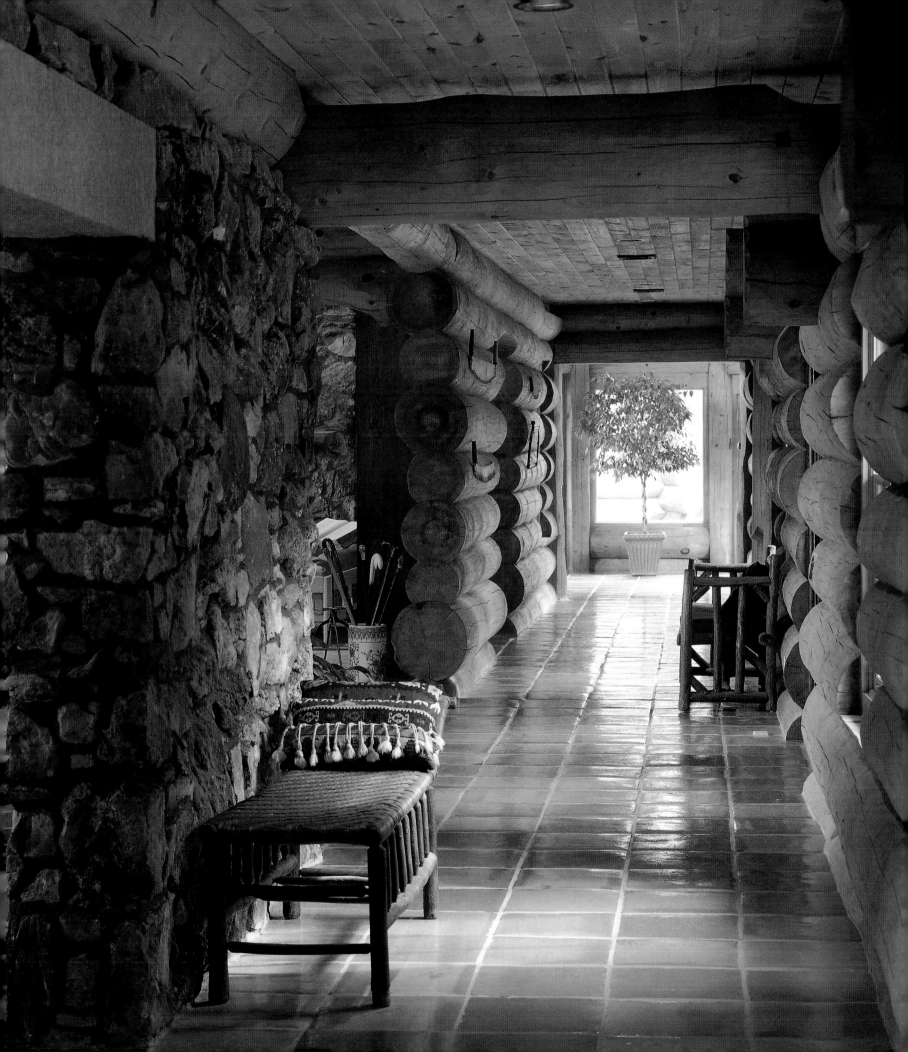

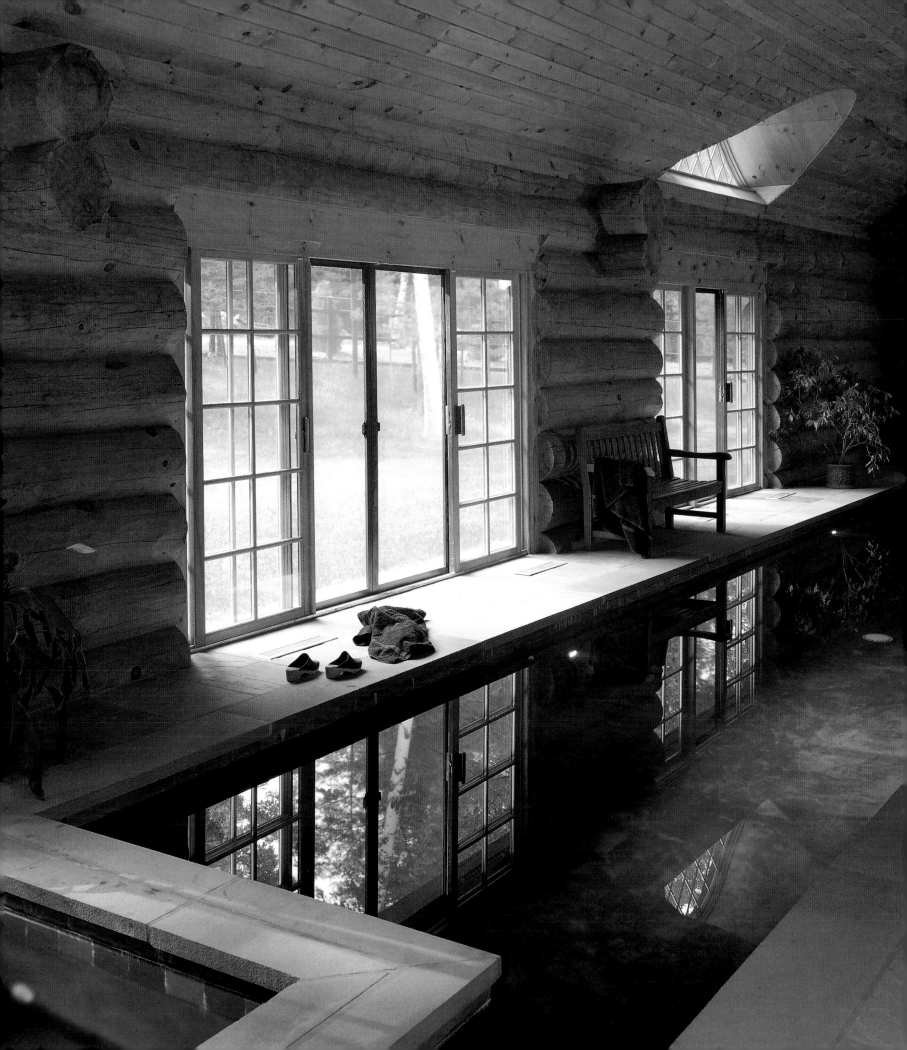

from wandering through the intriguing layout or walking and biking the trails on the 65-acre property, the owners can use the exercise room, lap pool, and spa.

The well-equipped exercise room is located a half-level above the garage, with windows optimally placed to look down on a valley. Behind and a half-level down from the exercise room is a lap pool that opens onto a private courtyard. The room's blue stone flooring complements the room's white pine log walls and plank ceilings. Three sets of nine-foot-wide glass doors, topped by eyebrow windows, bathe the room in light. The windows' triple insulation keeps the room comfortable.

Humidity control is a high priority, since moisture generated by a pool can damage exposed and structural wood. To remove humidity from the air efficiently, Martin used a complex Dry-O-Tron dehumidifying system. Heat generated by the system's motor does double duty by warming the pool, so the water is always ready for a swim.

Fitting natural details in the simple room save it from being Spartan and reinforce the aura of a rustic retreat.

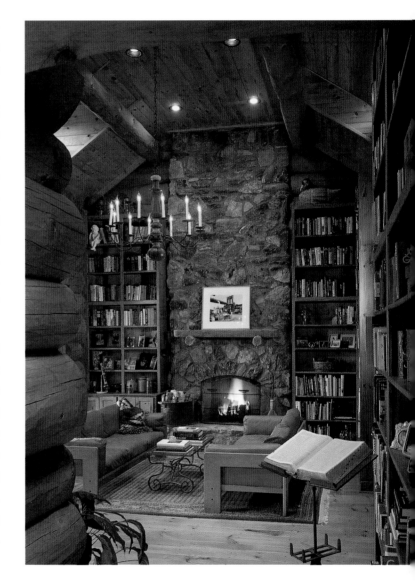

Navigating Body and Soul

THE NINEVAH BEACH HOUSE

NO BOOK ON FITNESS AND HOMES would be complete without a mention of the beach house. Whether it's a summer house or multi-seasonal residence, a beach house by its very existence promotes fitness, encouraging a quick dip in the frothy waves and long, muscle-toning walks on the sand.

The sea and sky propel the design of the Ninevah Beach House, designed by Louise Braverman. The house appears to rush head-long into the Long Island Sound. Its design is all about its site, a 30-foot-high bluff over-looking the sound. Set on Sag Harbor's high-est elevation, it perches on the bluff as if ready to spring into the water. Its slightly angled yet continuous roof, reinforced by its four-and-a-half-foot overhang, gently moves upward and outward toward the water, rein-forcing a visual relationship with the sea.

This relationship is further amplified by the linear path from the street to the water through a series of architectural volumes twist-ing and turning slightly as they progress from the entry stair, through the two-story stair tower, out and down the stairs at the bluff to the sand and sea. "The house is all about move-ment," said Braverman, "lots of movement up and down stairs, indoors and outdoors."

Although the home's roots lie in the tradition of Sag Harbor, it draws inspiration from contemporary California beach-front towns. It was built for a client who was

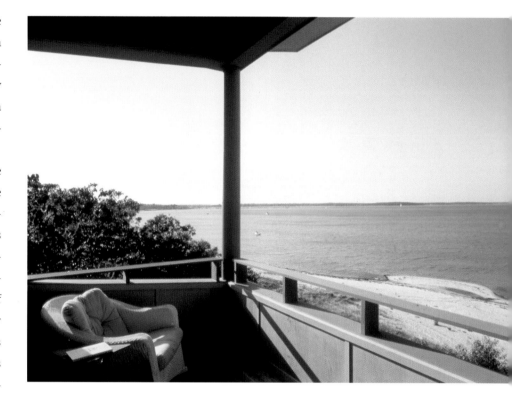

ABOVE and RIGHT: A glimmering expanse of bay beckons from Long Island Sound and the home's outdoor step seem to hurry toward its waters. Although the home is located in Long Island, New York, its spare elemental approach lends the eastern island some of California's breezy design flair.

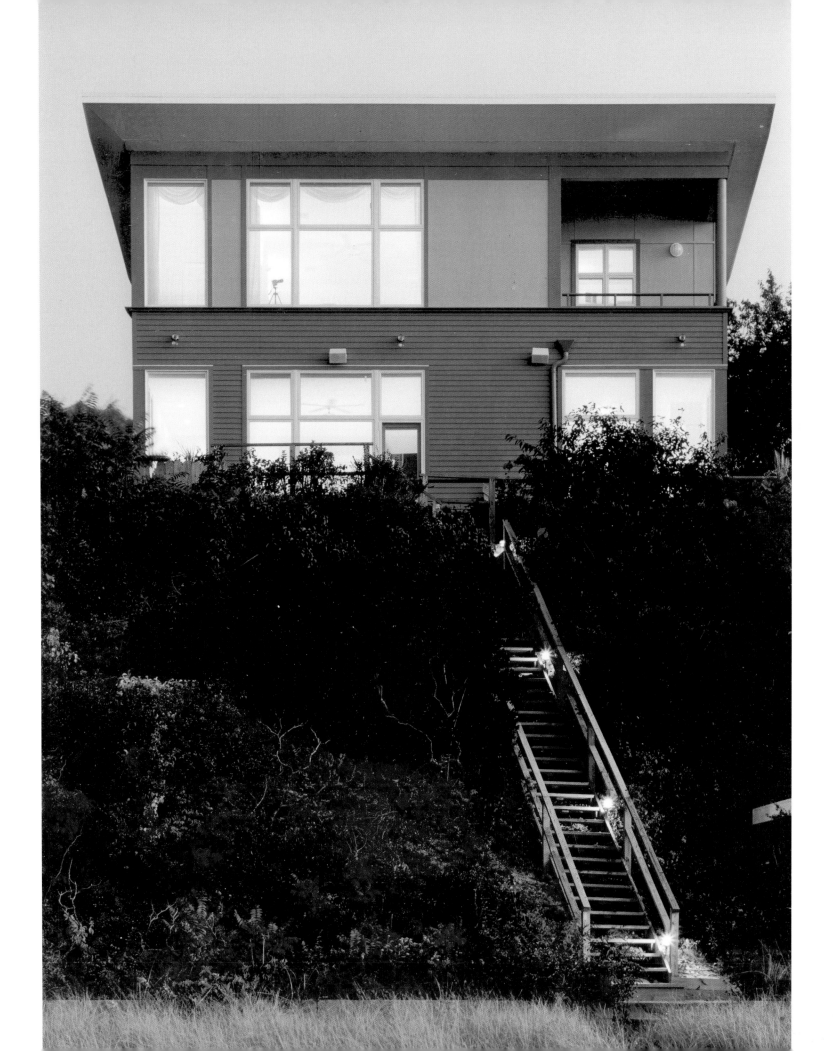

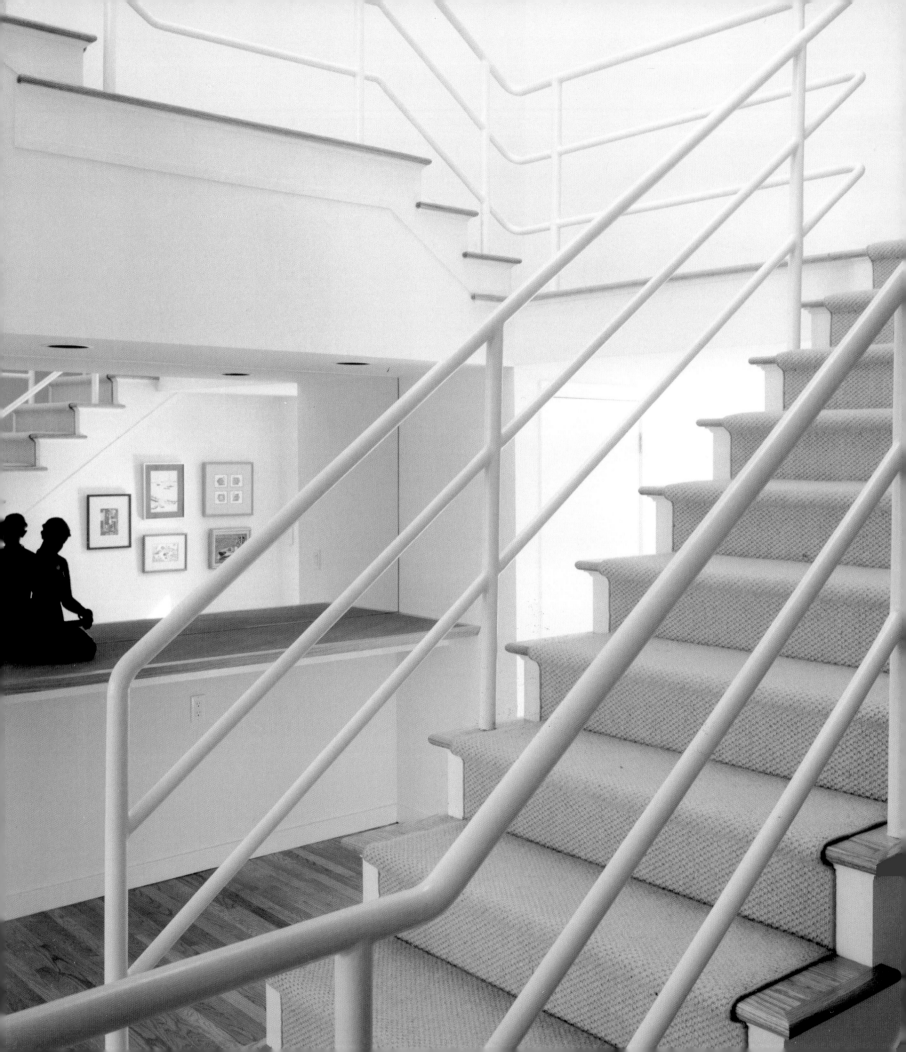

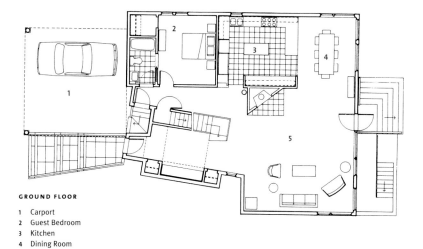

GROUND FLOOR

1   Carport
2   Guest Bedroom
3   Kitchen
4   Dining Room
5   Living Area

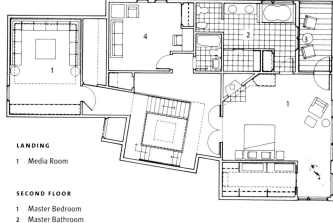

LANDING

1   Media Room

SECOND FLOOR

1   Master Bedroom
2   Master Bathroom
3   Balcony
4   Study

LEFT and RIGHT: An overhead clerestory bathes the stairs in natural light and draws the climber upwards. The stair angles are all about movement—from the Sound's waters to the master bedroom, which offers the best view of the Sound.

raised in southern California, likes the outdoors, and enjoys fishing. According to Braverman, her client "wanted to feel nature, to look into the front door and see the sea beyond. That was a priority." Open the front door of this blue-gray cedar house and you can see the sea beyond and the sky above through an overhead clerestory.

It also seemed fitting that a homeowner who liked to gaze at the heavens through a telescope should have windows designed to give a panoramic, 180-degree view of the sea. In the master bedroom, expansive windows are flanked by smaller windows to widen the view further.

The home is all about a visual communion with the waves, whether you're moving horizontally through the house from the street to the sea or vertically up the angled stair tower toward the clerestory light. Braverman describes the stairs as doughnut shaped.

"You go to a partial level, can see views of the sea and then go higher and you can see more," she said. The stairs culminate at the master bedroom with its expansive view of prime fishing waters.

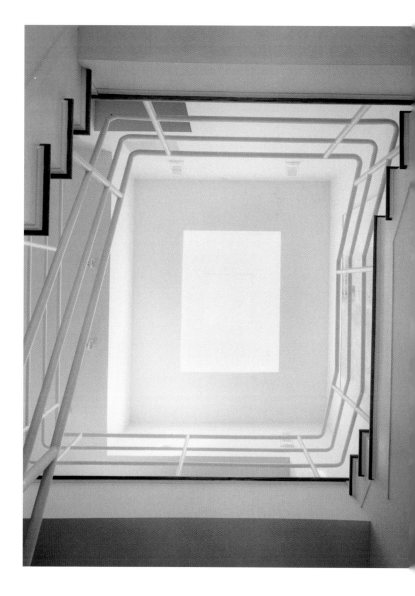

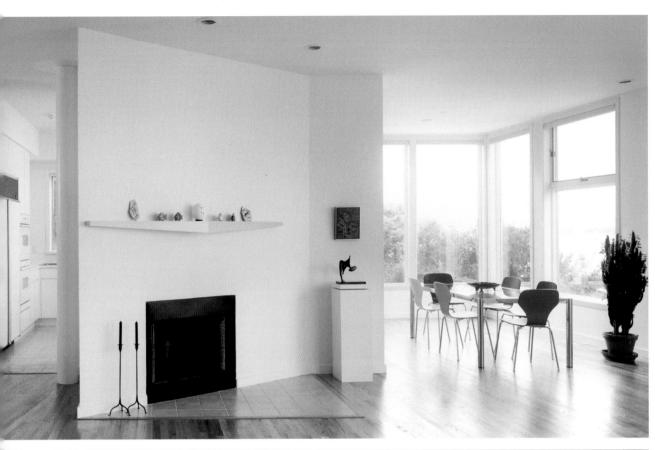

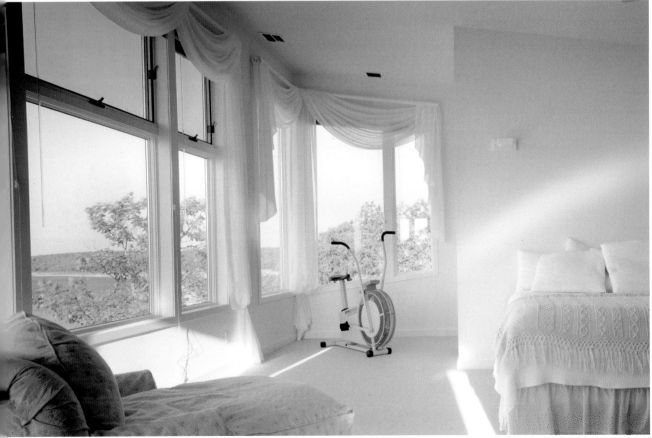

LEFT, ABOVE and BELOW, and RIGHT: The owner of this home wanted to see nature and the house offers expansive views to satisfy that request, from the dining room (above left) to the master bedroom, where an exercise bicycle (below left) takes full advantage of the Sound's prime fishing waters and a telescope (right) is set to track the constellations.

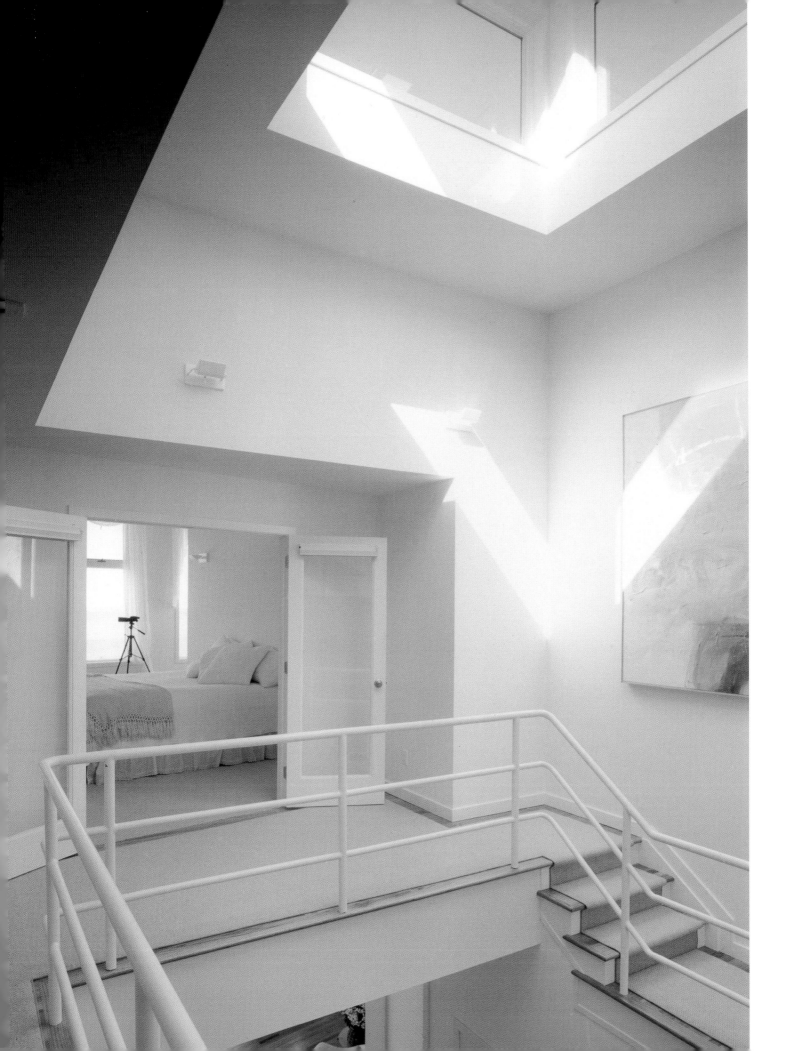

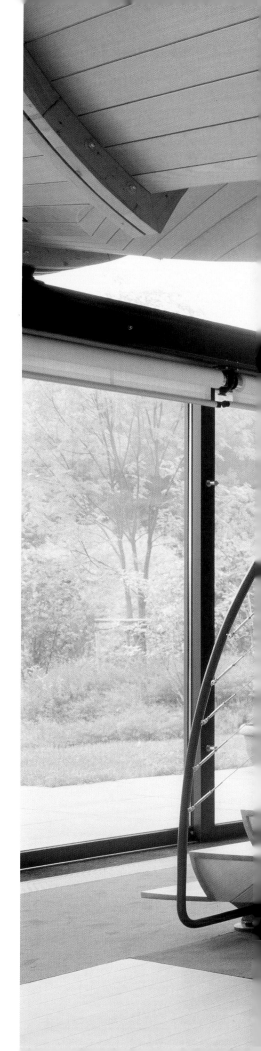

Structuring Sport

THE SPINE HOUSE

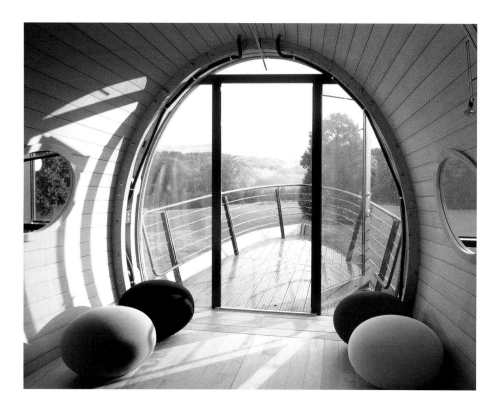

THE SPINE HOUSE, BUILT BY the British architect Sir Nicholas Grimshaw with Mark Bryden and Martin Wood, incorporates three elements of the high fit home: interesting stairs that are expressly designed to lead to a unique vantage point, a splayed layout that encourages walking, and two specific exercise features—a squash and tennis court. Its very design epitomizes balance, the basis of physical and mental health.

The Spine House was the first private residential project to be designed by Grimshaw. After he built a factory for the owners, residents

ABOVE: One of the rewards for climbing through the intriguing spine of this home is the view of the mature lime tree from the bridge. **RIGHT:** The high-tech space-age quality of the stairs designed to define this German home draws the climber upward, as surely as if the climber was beamed up to a spaceship. **OVER:** The spine is the defining feature of this spacious home, connecting the public ground-floor spaces with the more private second-floor area.

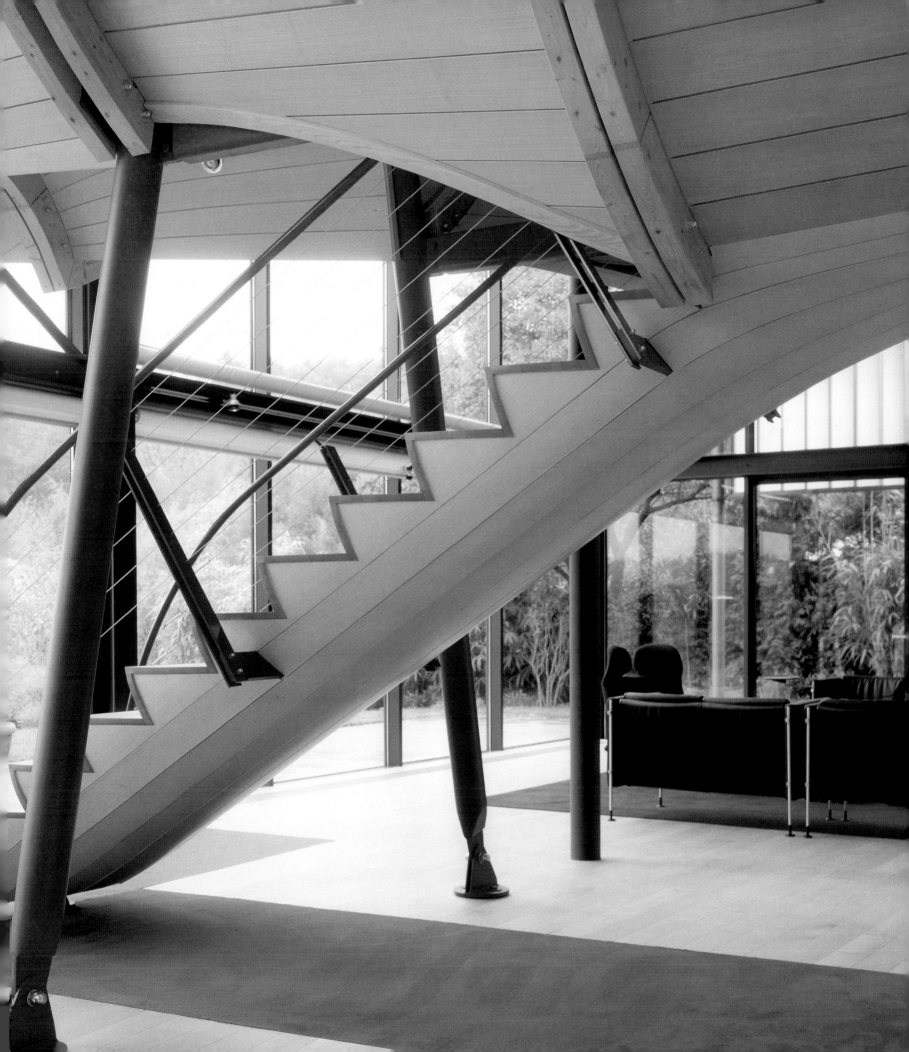

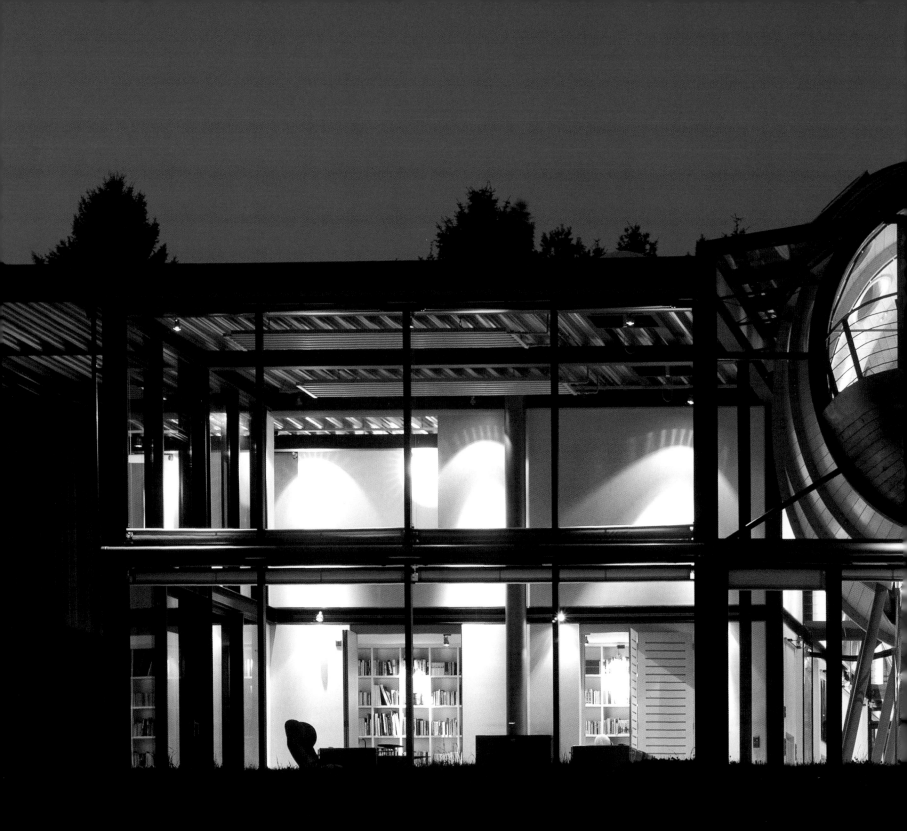

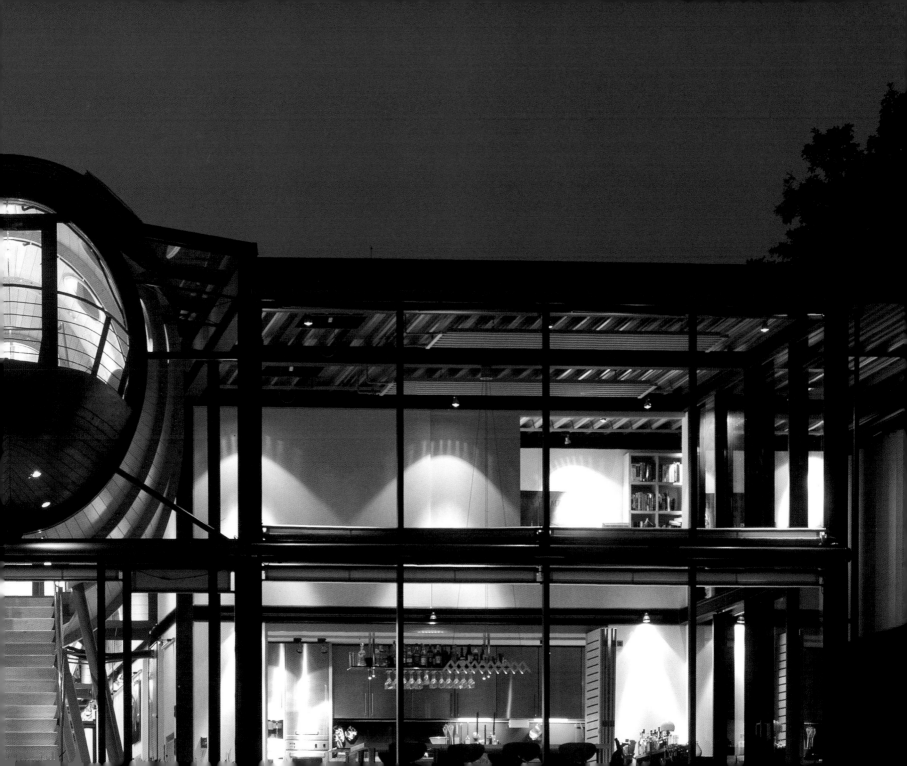

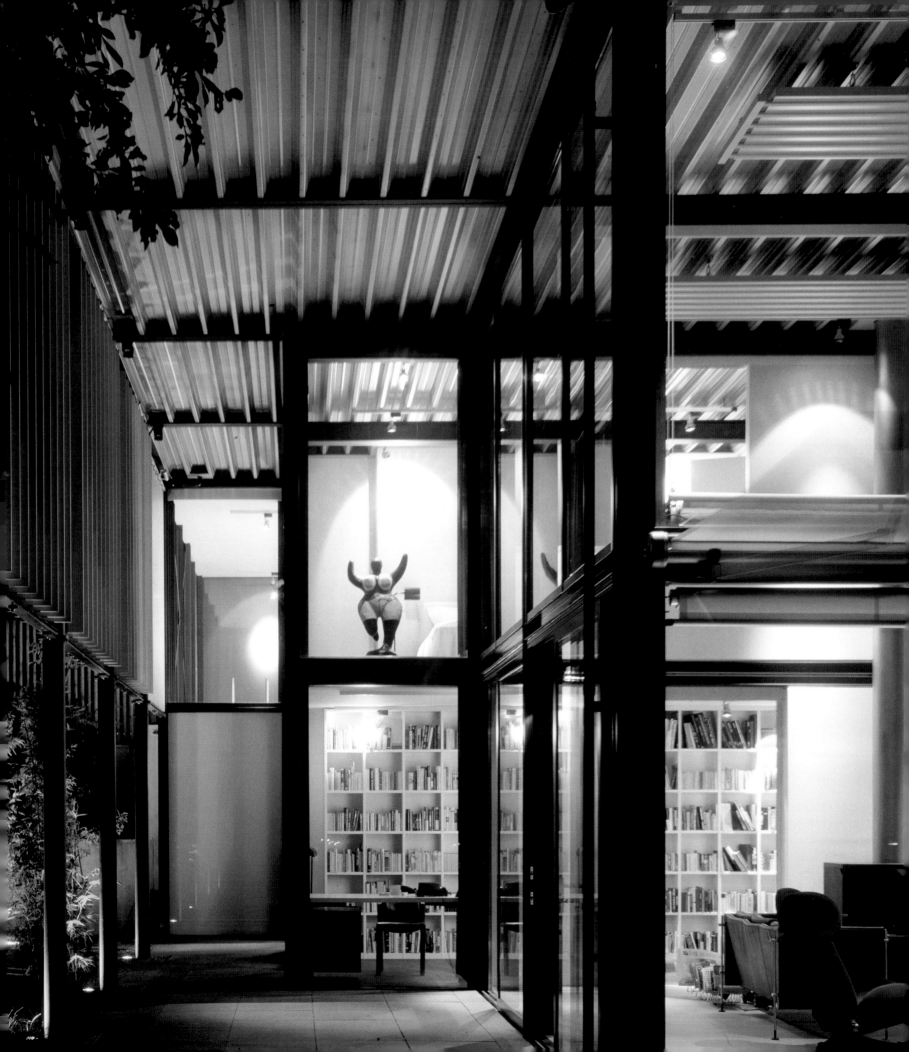

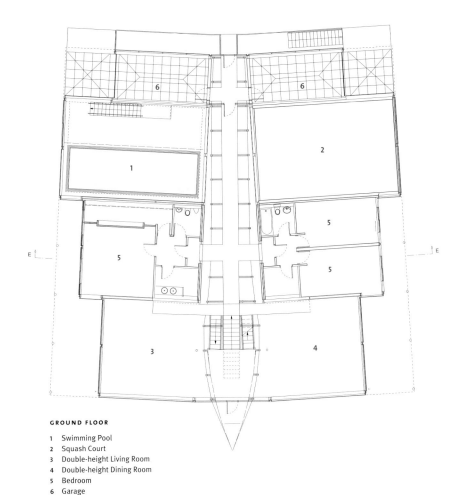

GROUND FLOOR

1 Swimming Pool
2 Squash Court
3 Double-height Living Room
4 Double-height Dining Room
5 Bedroom
6 Garage

LEFT: While the curves of the spine delineate the building, the rest is strictly rectilinear, perhaps in homage to the factory that the architect first designed for the couple living in this house. The defining central spine skews the home's rectangular views.

launched. The property is divided into two freestanding wings of accommodation. Its strict rectilinear form is halved by a long curvilinear "spine" pointing toward the south.

In the house as built, the spine has become the defining feature of the design. It is an interior in its own right, with a split-level sitting room and an external "cockpit" viewpoint. The spine does not have to provide any structural support for the building. It does not act simply as a mediating space between the wings but forces them apart, splaying the house as the land drops away toward the south. The splaying, which carries through the main façade, skews what might otherwise be rectangular living spaces, creating diagonal views throughout the house.

Internally, the spine runs the length of the second floor, elevated on angled steel legs (painted red). The full height space underneath enables the occupants to circulate among the closed spaces on the ground floor, such as the squash-tennis court and swimming pool. Lit by natural daylight filtered through the gaps on either side of the spine, it also functions as a private art gallery.

Walking through the spine, a visitor is conscious of a bright spot of light and the glowing landscape at its end. Although you enter at the ground floor, by the time you reach the vantage point, you are perched at the high end of the house. That vantage point was designed to focus on a mature lime tree.

The building is widest along the street elevation, narrowing toward the garden, thus affording south-facing views to the rooms behind the front living area (bedrooms on

of Cologne, Germany, the couple asked him to design them a home on sloping meadowland with distant views of Cologne.

Grimshaw, Bryden, and Wood devised the architectural concept for the Spine House in 1996. When Bryden and Wood formed their own practice, Bryden Wood Associates, Grimshaw invited them to run the project on a daily basis.

The house was designed for a family whose factory makes the plastic components for motorbikes, racing cars, and robots. With its boat and airplane imagery, the building seems so animated that parts of it might suddenly be

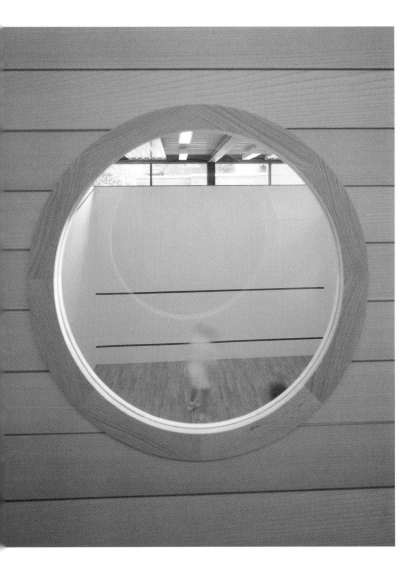

the second floor; studies on the ground floor) as the wings step inward. It also opens out downward on a north-south axis to reveal a two-story structure sunk into the landscape. The roof remains level: a single flat plane, save for the zinc-clad form of the spine.

Toward the south, the spine proceeds into an open-plan living and dining area, with a double-height glazed façade. It pictures this façade with its nose, providing a viewpoint over the landscape. The living/dining area is accessible from the ground floor by way of an open staircase that is aligned with the double doors leading out into the garden.

The spine was handcrafted in eight individual laminated rib sections supporting timber cladding that is visible from both inside and out. These were bolted together on site. The American ash timbers add an organic note to a palette of otherwise industrial materials—steel frame, glass cladding, aluminum louvers.

Behind the house, the squash-tennis court and swimming pool offer two different takes on fitness that seem as balanced as the home's design.

LEFT: From one of the portholes of the home's spine, you can see the squash-tennis court in which blurry figures rev up their metabolism by chasing the ball. RIGHT: The spine, handcrafted from American ash timbers, also offers views of the other rooms in the home. It has a ship-like quality, imbuing the basic shapes of the house with spirit and a shade of irony.

high fit home

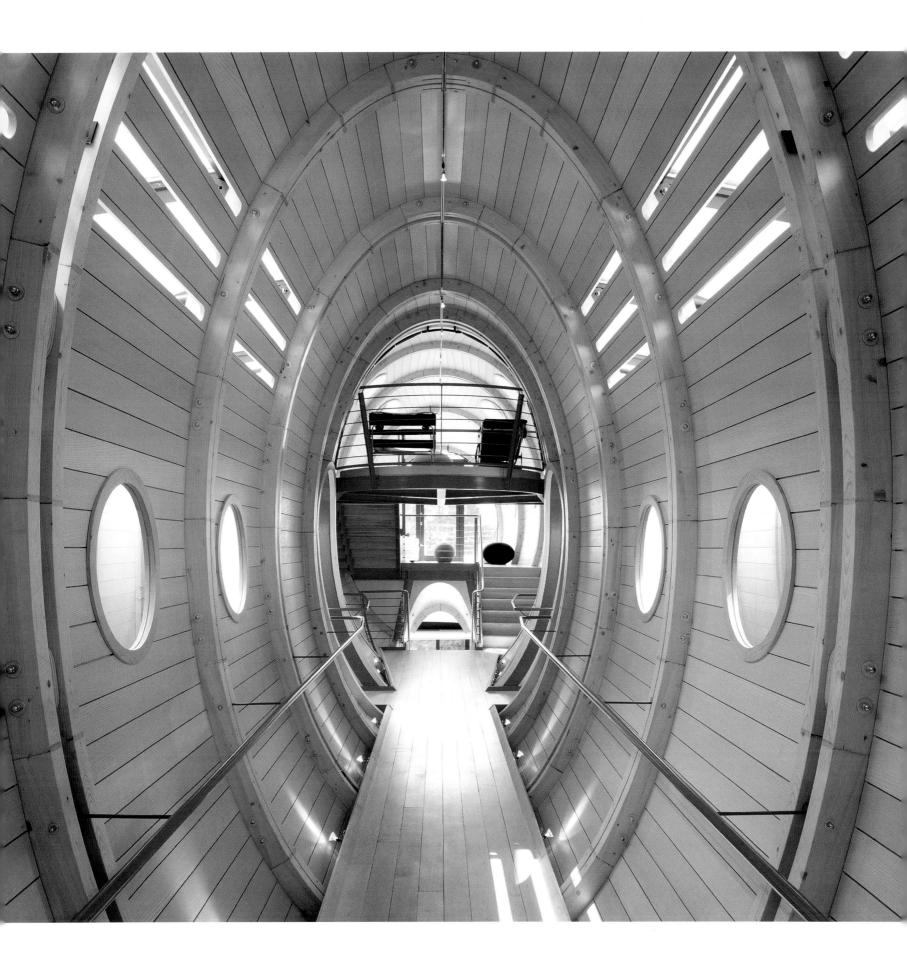

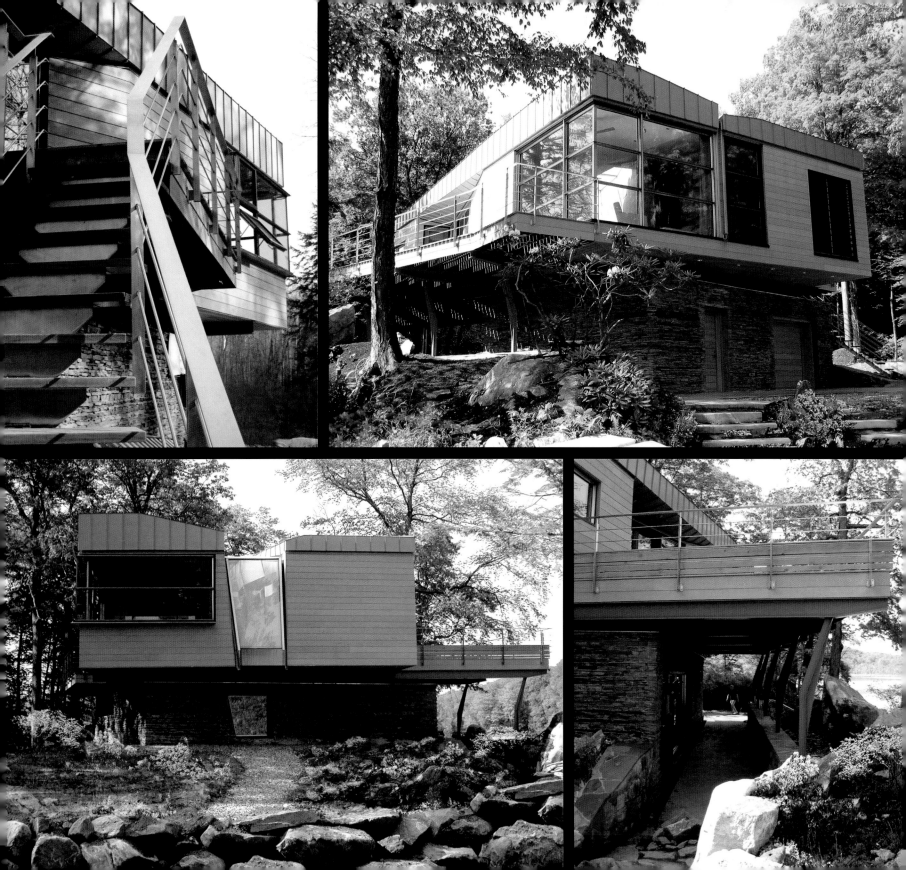

Integrating Fitness into Landscape

THE GIPSY TRAIL HOUSE

LEFT: A low-maintenance zinc roof and cedar siding, treated only with bleaching stain, ensures that there's time for outdoor fun and that one day this home will blend into the lakeside wood and rocks.
BELOW: A gym with a view of a placid lake is all the inspiration this suburban family needs to practice yoga and lift weights. The family also likes to flex their muscles by biking, canoeing on the lake, and skiing.

FOR CITY DWELLERS, there's often a social aspect to going to the gym, but for family-focused suburbanites, bringing the gym to the home can be a more realistic goal than getting the person to the gym. For exercise to fit into a complex schedule of meshing priorities, working out needs to be an integral part of daily life.

While exercise was a priority, accessibility and privacy were the two most important homeowner requests that Winka Dubbledam faced when designing the Gipsy Trail House, which faces the Croton Reservoir in upstate New York. The homeowners, who she describes as super active and nature loving, wanted a living space that not only enabled them to work out but also to be comfortable walking from the gym into an outdoor shower or to a hot tub hidden in the rocks. "They definitely wanted a gym and a space where they could do yoga, from the very beginning," said Dubbledam, a principal at New York City's archi-tectonics.

To provide such privacy and freedom, the home's design was carefully integrated into the landscape, with its design and materials inspired by the terrain. About a fourth of the recessed ground floor is used for exercise space. Because of the way the house fits intimately into the landscape and the way the

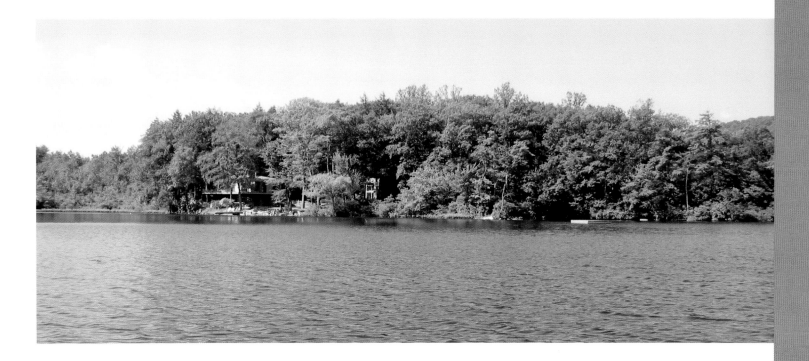

GROUND FLOOR

1 Gym
2 Guest Bedroom
3 Mudroom
4 Garage
5 Laundry Room
6 Guest Bath/Sauna
7 Pathways

SECOND FLOOR

1 Entrance
2 Sunroom
3 Study
4 Living Room
5 Kitchen
6 Dining Room
7 Master Bedroom
8 Master Bathroom
9 Deck

ground floor tucks under an expansive terrace, the gym's huge windows offer shimmering views of the lake while providing privacy. "The great thing about this house is that you can see the lake while you're working out, but boaters on the lake cannot see in," said Dubbledam.

Besides being outfitted with a glorious view, the gym contains mostly weights. It has ample space for yoga, which the homeowners practice when they are not biking, canoeing on the lake, or skiing. "One important idea that we developed the house around was a constant inside-outside connection, all year long," said Dubbledam.

To create more time for the fun-fit things in life, the house is as maintenance free as possible, with a zinc roof and cedar siding treated only with a bleaching oil. The treatment means the siding will automatically silver, ultimately blending the roof, stainless steel features, and ground floor of indigenous rock into one warm, natural gray. One day, the 3,000-square-foot house will blend into the landscape, whose elements it displaced. The window frames were made from afromosia, a strong hardwood, similar to teak.

The house's structural center resides in a centrally located core or armature, which integrates the kitchen, the bathrooms, the fireplace, the heating and cooling system, and a central music system. Where the roof

bends to meet the armature, glass panes take the place of the zinc roof in the form of a continuous skylight. As the sun completes its arc through the sky, the armature collects rays and disperses them throughout the house. Where the glass bends over to become wall at the end of the armature, a transparent shower room is suspended between the trees.

Tucked like a backpack over the two-car garage is the guesthouse, a simple, 1,500-square-foot version of the house, also crafted to honor and one day meld with its surroundings.

RIGHT: A centrally located armature integrates the bathrooms (above, left and right), the kitchen (below right and left), the fireplace, heating and cooling systems, and a central music system. Generous windows and glass doors help reinforce the inside-outside connection that the homeowners longed for.

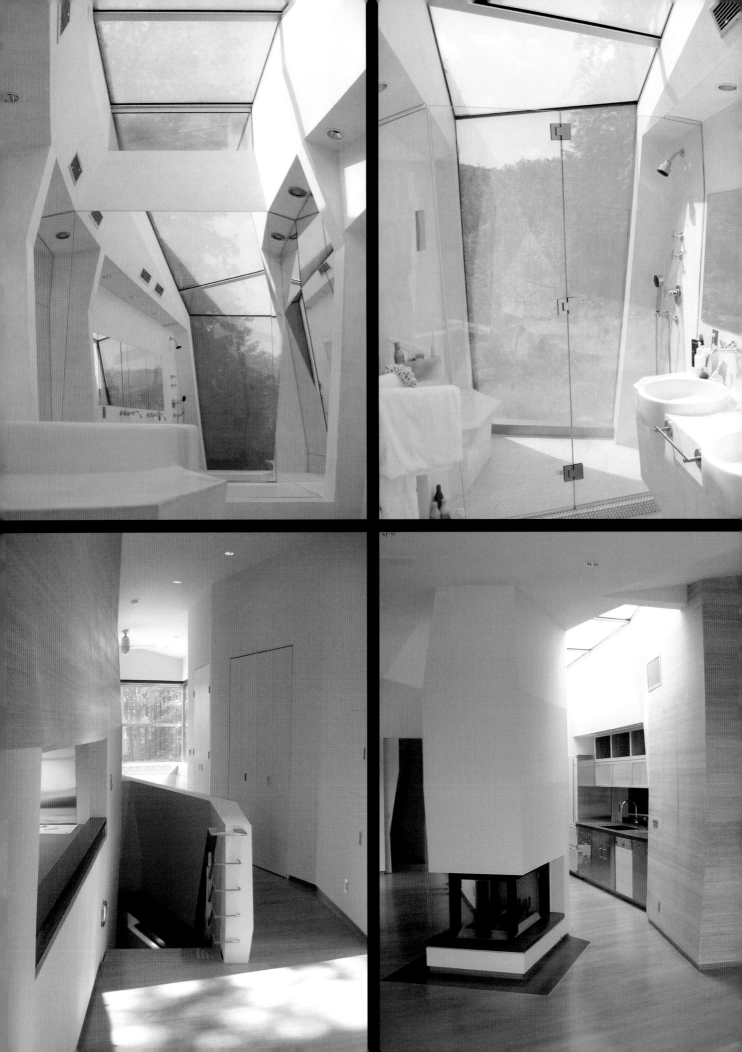

A Family Retreat on Track

THE MOUNTAIN HOUSE

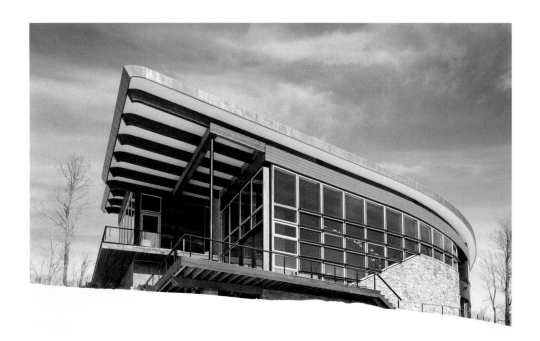

DEVELOPED AS A FAMILY RETREAT and ski lodge by Graftworks, the Mountain House in Stratton, Vermont, captures visual elements associated with the sport and benefits admirably from the technology used to create and laminate snow skis. Located on a 150-acre mountainous, wooded site, the house follows the curving contour of the land, maximizing views in two directions. The diagram of the house grew from the idea of movement and threshold. By following the flow of the land, the long side of the house captures the horizon with views of distant Mount Snow, while the ends of the house inflect toward nearby Stratton Mountain.

ABOVE and RIGHT: The construction of the Mountain House in Stratton, Vermont, follows the contours of the land on which it's built. A winter ski lodge built for a large family, its design also mimics the snow tracks left by skis. The home's 150-acre site offers opportunities for hiking and walking. An on-site tennis court with stunning mountain views provides the possibility of exercise in warmer weather.

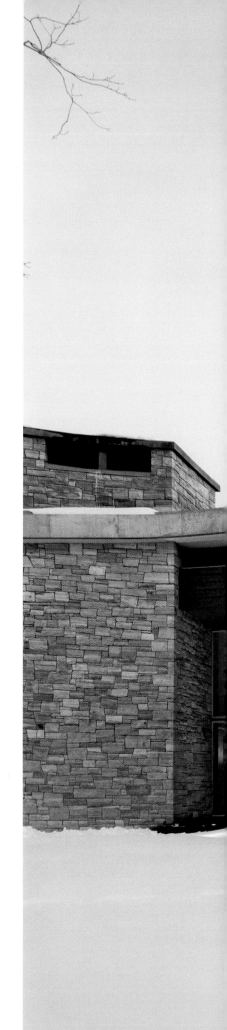

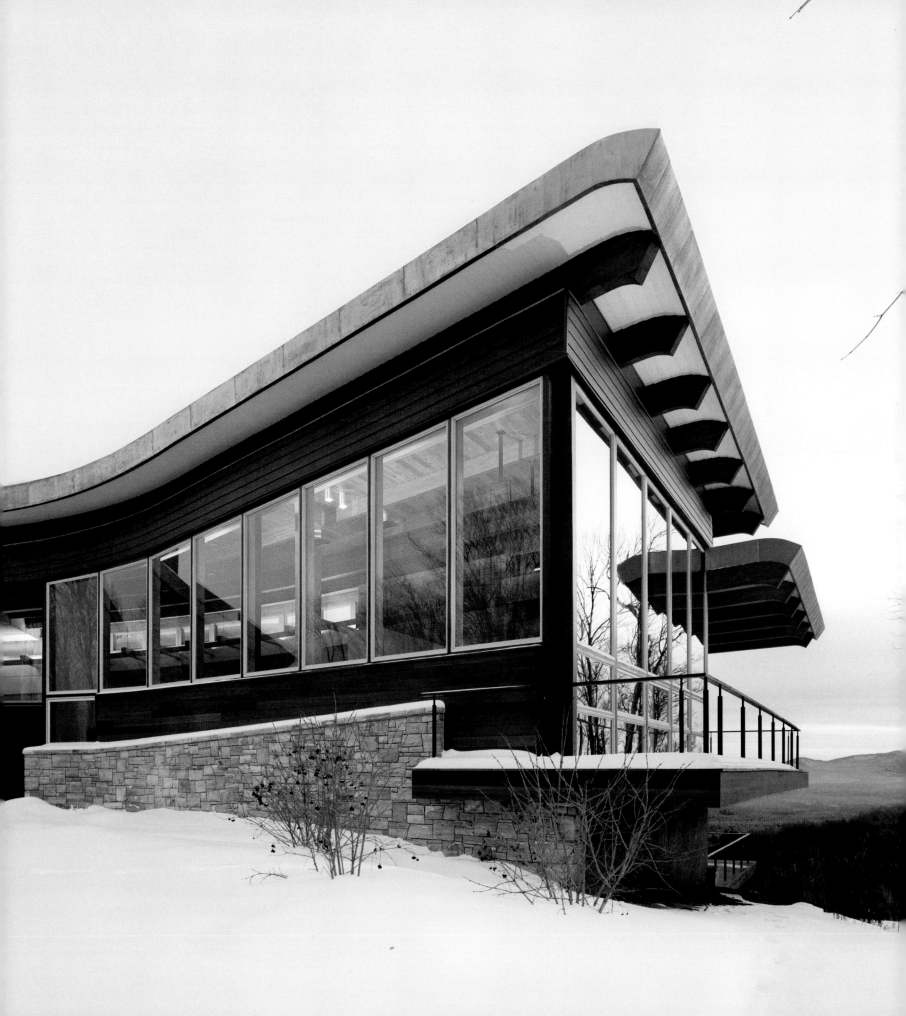

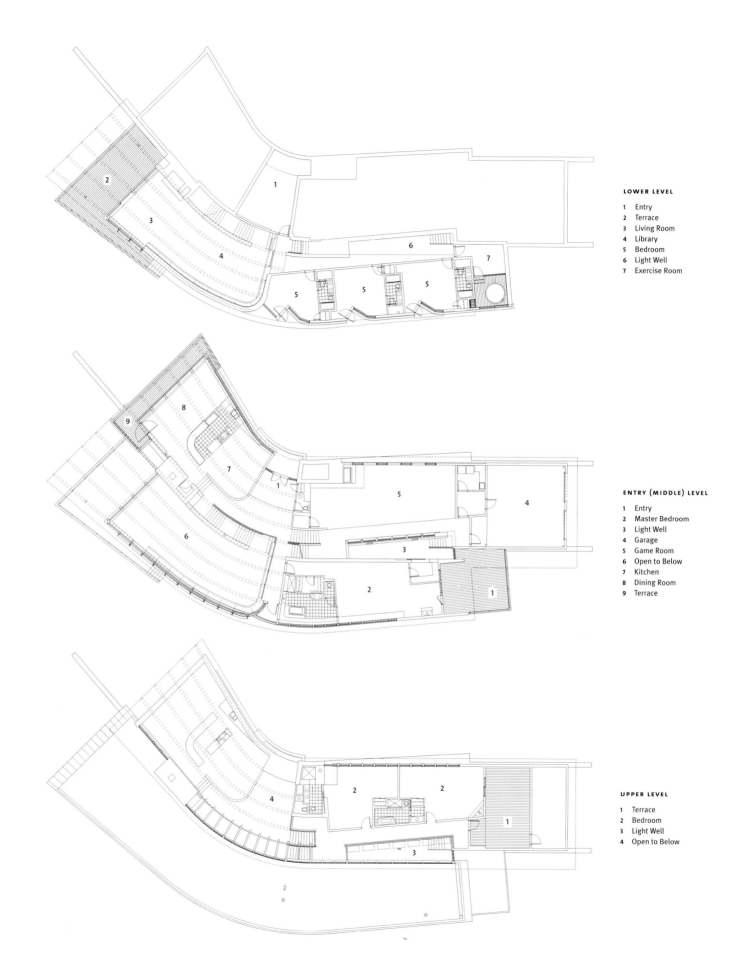

LOWER LEVEL

1 Entry
2 Terrace
3 Living Room
4 Library
5 Bedroom
6 Light Well
7 Exercise Room

ENTRY (MIDDLE) LEVEL

1 Entry
2 Master Bedroom
3 Light Well
4 Garage
5 Game Room
6 Open to Below
7 Kitchen
8 Dining Room
9 Terrace

UPPER LEVEL

1 Terrace
2 Bedroom
3 Light Well
4 Open to Below

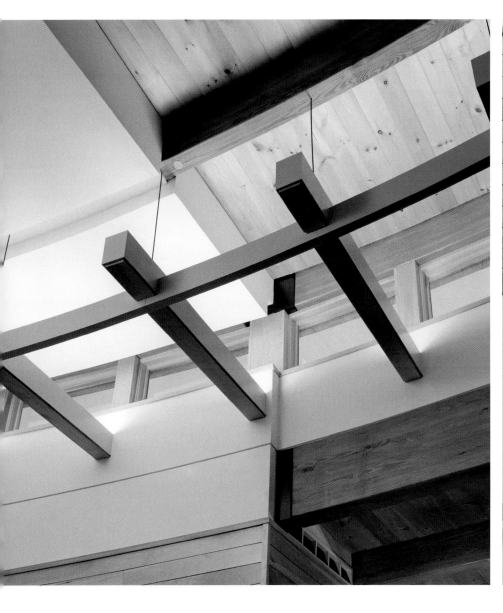

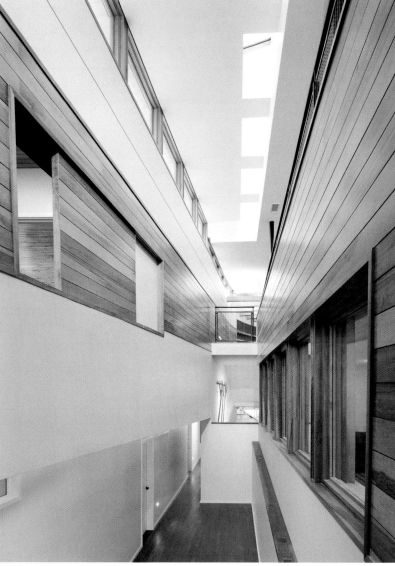

ABOVE, LEFT and RIGHT: Flowing lines are evident in the interior as well as the exterior of this ski house with various levels of communal activities divided among floors, inviting the frequent use of stairs. When asked if they wanted an elevator, the homeowners declined. A house centered on physical activity should not skip the benefits of stair climbing, they said.

The interior of the house is conceived as a landscape with varying sections. The house is organized into two interlocking strands that terrace with the section of the mountain. A clerestory runs the length between the two strands, washing the interior with light while continuously referring to the horizon. Both strands slope and curve from the rear of the house to the front. Bedrooms and more private spaces are organized in the rear of the house, where the ceiling heights are lower and the views more restricted; living and dining spaces occupy the front of the house, where the ceil-

ing ascends to a height of 18 feet and the views are most expansive. The house seems to perch on the mountainside, with one end firmly secured by the terrain; while the living and dining rooms appear ready to take wing.

The circulation of the house originates in the zone between the two strands and connects the two terraces. Different speeds of circulation are distributed throughout the house: slow where the space is dilated (group activities or living) and fast where the space is compressed (individual activities or rest). At the rear of the house, the circulation spills

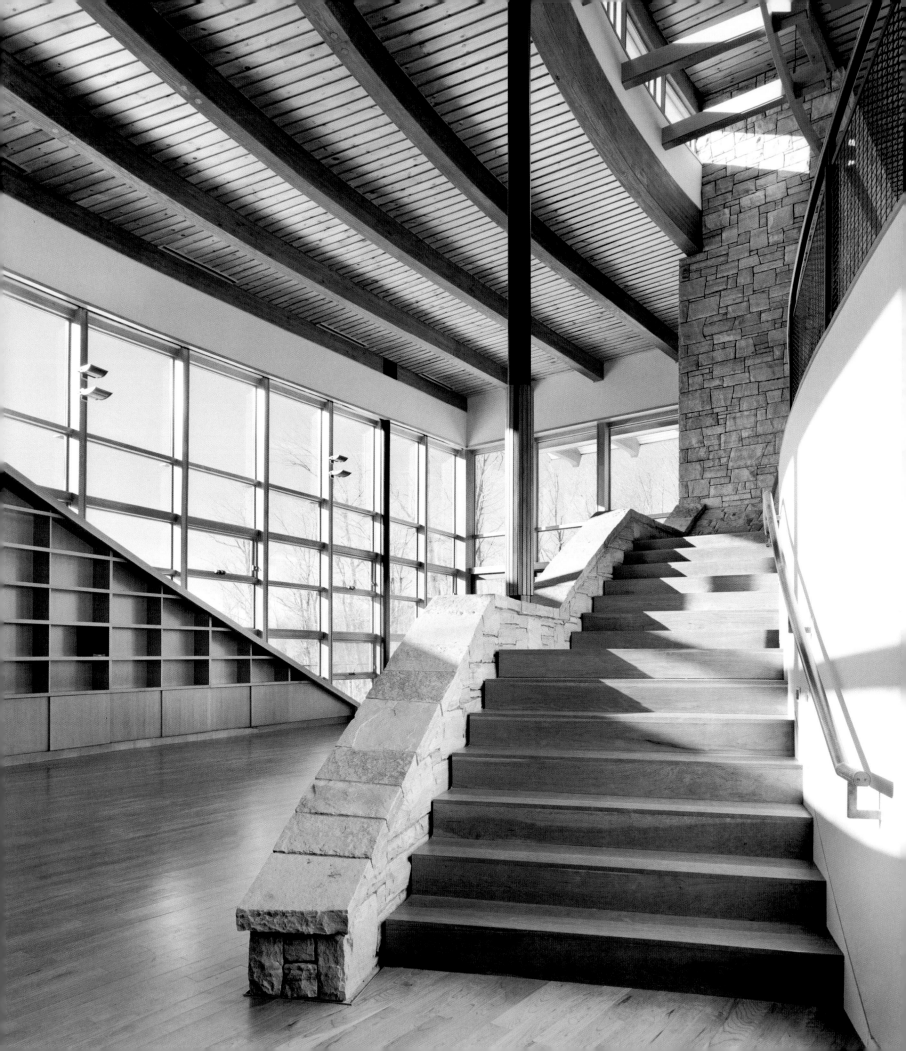

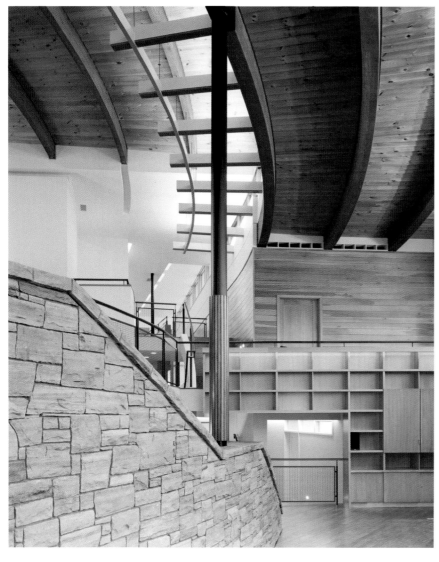

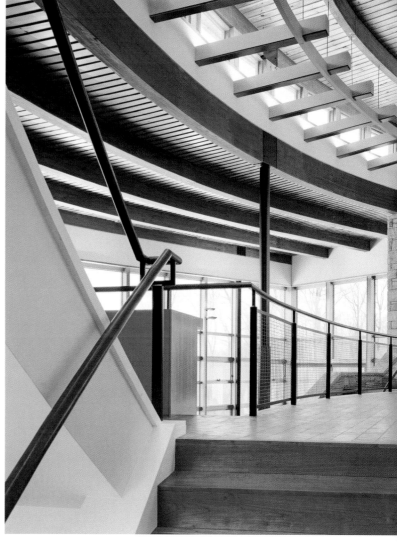

LEFT: Although the home's design is lean, clean, and linear, there's room for captivating details, such as this built-in bookshelf on an incline, reminiscent of a ski slope. ABOVE, LEFT and RIGHT: Wooden slats that evoke tracks help express the home's sense of movement, while a fine mesh rail makes the stairs safer without obscuring the view.

into a light well that acts as a communicating space between the entry level and lower-level bedrooms, and the children's game room and exercise room.

"The house is really like a journey," said architect Lawrence Blough of the many ways it's possible to move through and around the house he designed with his fellow Graftworks principal John Henle.

With the game room down a half level from some bedrooms and up a half level from others, Blough offered to install an elevator, but the homeowners felt it was out of character for a home centered on so much physi-

cal activity. They not only wanted to use the stairs but requested seating be included on a series of stair balconies so guests can read and socialize there.

The home's lower bedrooms have an exterior terrace with direct access to the logging trails that crisscross the mountain. These trails lead to tennis courts 250 yards away. Terraced into the mountain, the tennis courts offer a stunning view of Bromley Mountain.

The striated organization of the house was inspired by the technology used in the lamination and manufacture of snow skis. Pine glue-laminated beams span parallel to

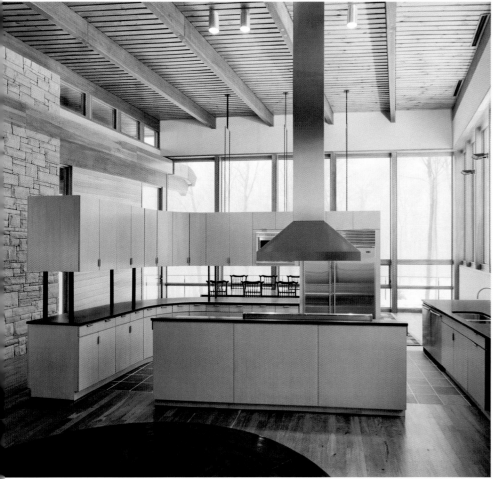

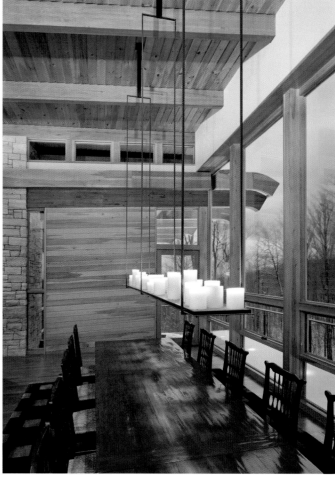

the length of the house, as opposed to conventional perpendicular framing, intensifying the ruled effect. Supported by columns hung at intermediate joints from concealed girders in the ceiling plenum, the beams were fabricated in 25-feet-long segments and then organized into continuous lines of structure.

Exterior materials include stone chimneys of local quartzite, cedar tongue-and-groove siding, lead-coated fascias, cambara decks, and slate walks. The home's circulation, access to the outside, and stairs all provide visual references to ski trails and inspire motion.

ABOVE, LEFT and RIGHT: A comfortable kitchen and dining room promote a sense of happy gathering. Small spaces to sit and read, some of which are found on stair landings, offer a place to enjoy privacy or share conversation. RIGHT: Waiting for its shelves to be filled to the brim with books, this comfortable room provides a place to sit and dream after skiing.

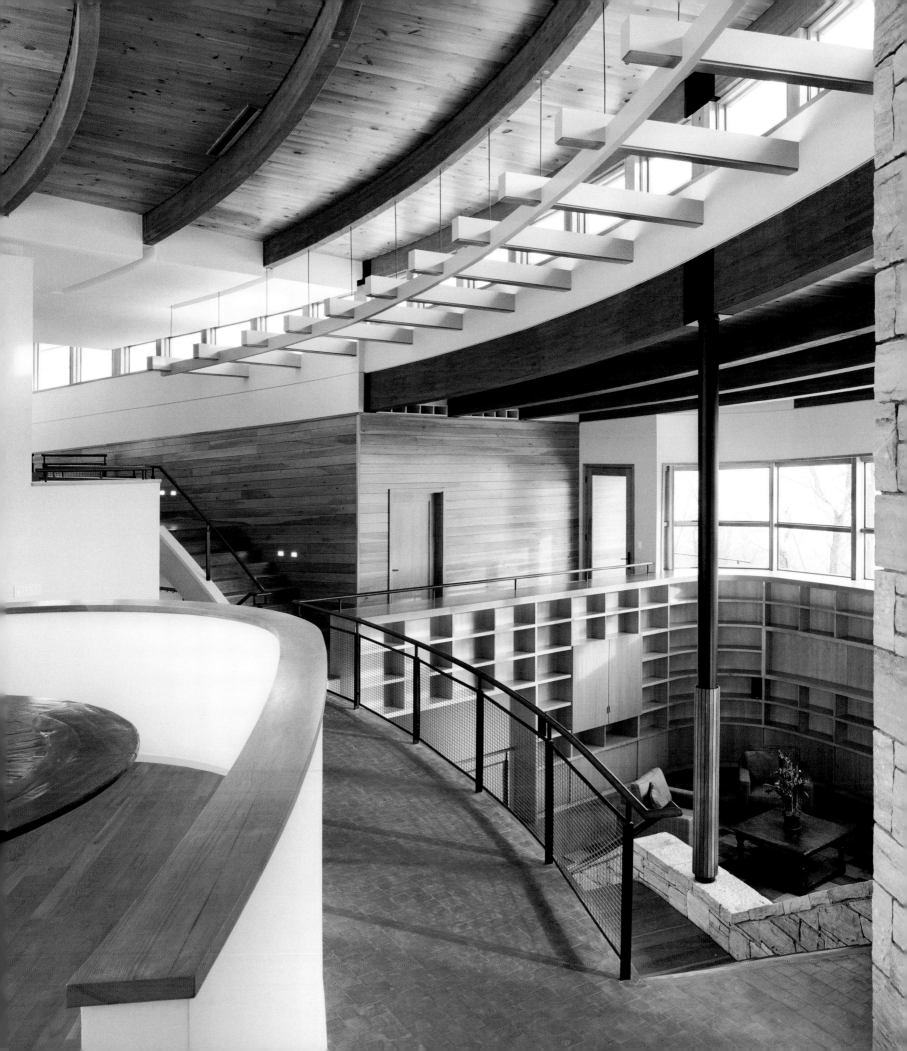

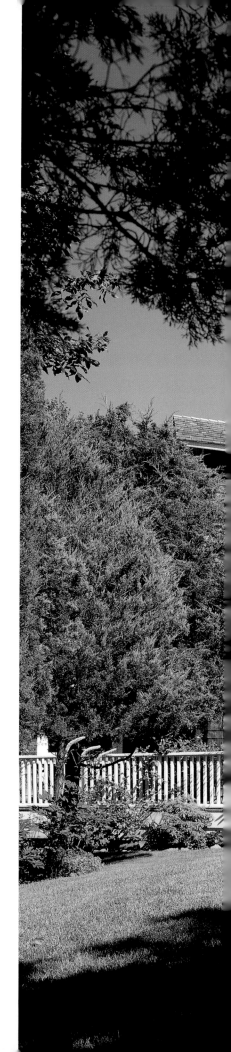

Making Fitness Playful

THE CARRIAGE HOUSE

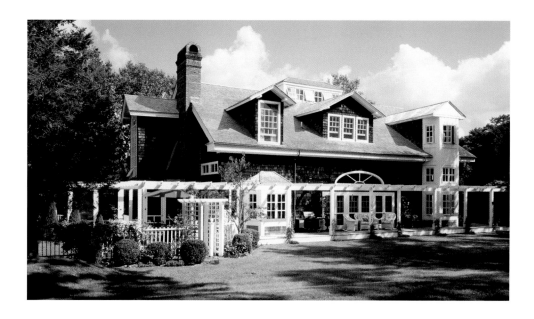

THE CARRIAGE HOUSE, a 15-year-long reno-vation of a former stable, has found more than one way to focus the unbridled energy of one young family. With three growing kids and active parents, the house is constantly on the move. Its breezy, open design anticipates spending time outdoors, extending the out-doors in and the indoors out, with the deck and pergola acting as the transition. Outdoors the yards are broken into several designated activity areas: the fenced-in swimming pool, plus a small vegetable garden.

The first phase of the renovation addressed the core of the house, which had never evolved from its original purpose—housing horses, carriages, tack-equipment, and several stablehands. The plumbing, heating, electrical

ABOVE and RIGHT: The active family who lives in this Long Island home plays basketball, croquet, tennis volleyball, golf, surfs, and swims. Their home—a renovated stable, which featured stalls for horses—is surrounded by areas designated for energy-expending activities.

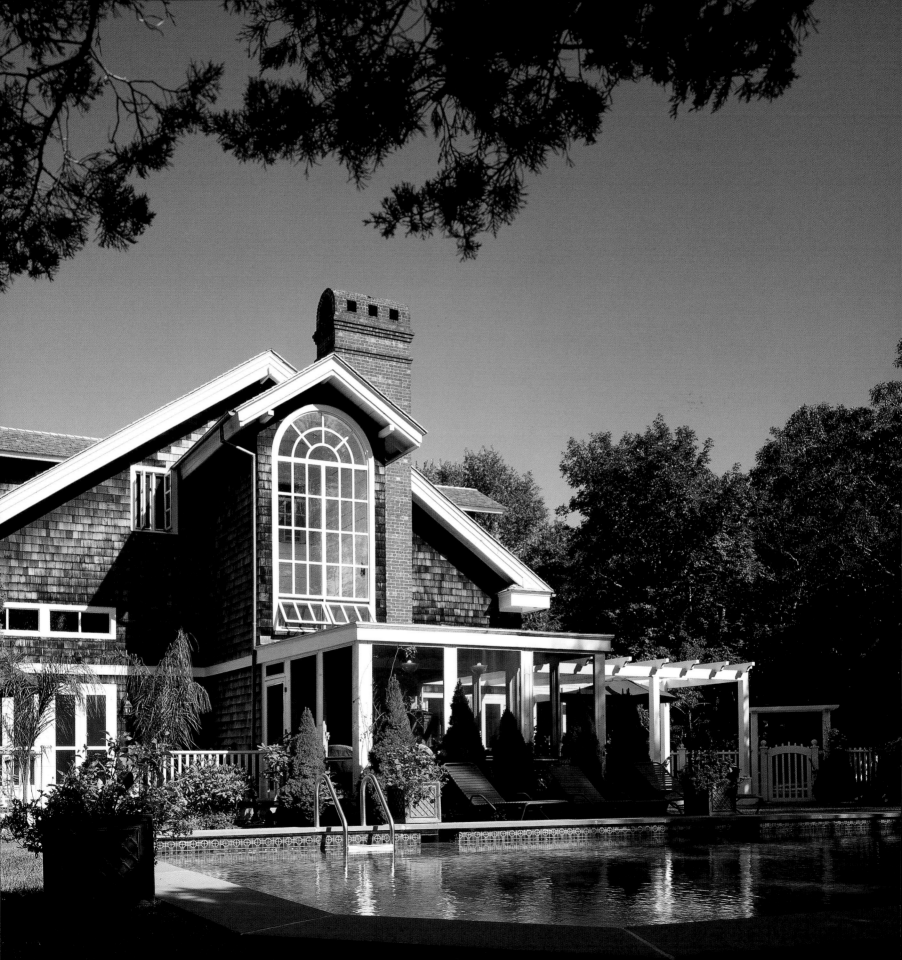

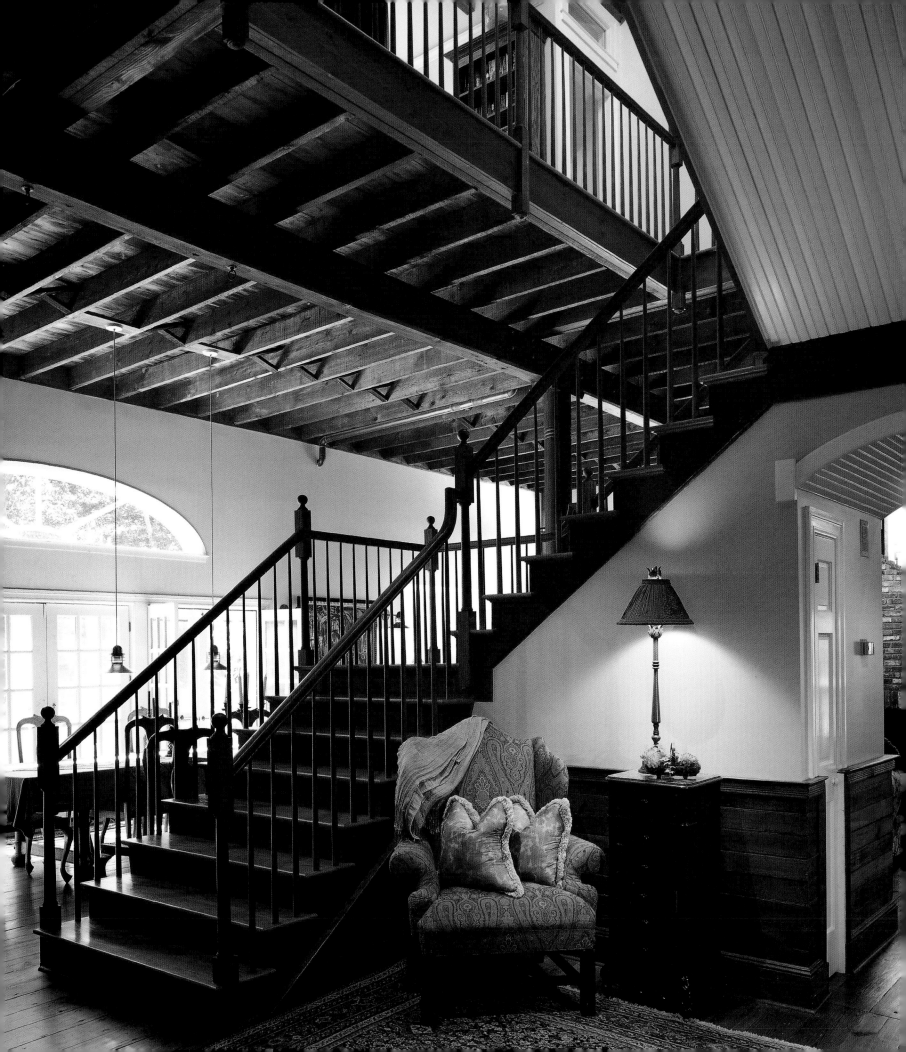

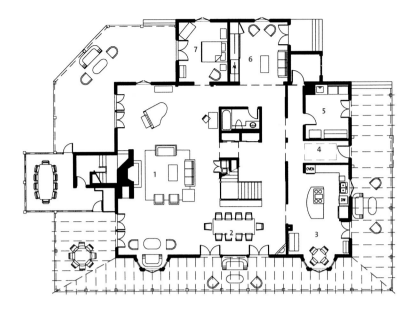

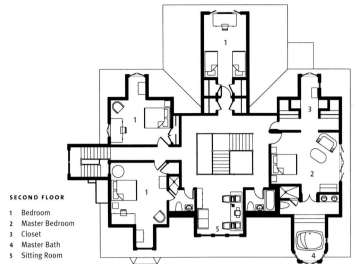

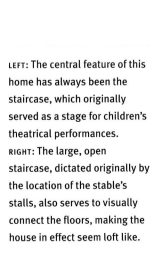

LEFT: The central feature of this home has always been the staircase, which originally served as a stage for children's theatrical performances.
RIGHT: The large, open staircase, dictated originally by the location of the stable's stalls, also serves to visually connect the floors, making the house in effect seem loft like.

installation, reshingling, and replacement of windows was completed in the early 1990s.

In this home on the south shore of Long Island, the central feature has always been a staircase. The stair defines the space, dividing it into quadrants: the living area, the music area, the dining area, and the summer seating. Surrounding the two sides of the central space are the stalls, now converted into a kitchen, mudroom, family room, and guest bedroom. The family room has a full-height storage unit across its west wall, which houses the entertainment center as well as stores larger equipment such as surfboards, boogie boards, and sleds. The staircase encloses storage for tennis rackets and balls and also houses a secret clubhouse for the kids under the first landing. Life is focused around the stair, as it is both stairs and stage for the growing children, who liked to play and present plays on it.

"The first landing is four and a half feet wide," said Ethelind Coblin, "and the kids would do little skits up and down the stairs. When you're sitting in the living room you can look right up there and see the homemade

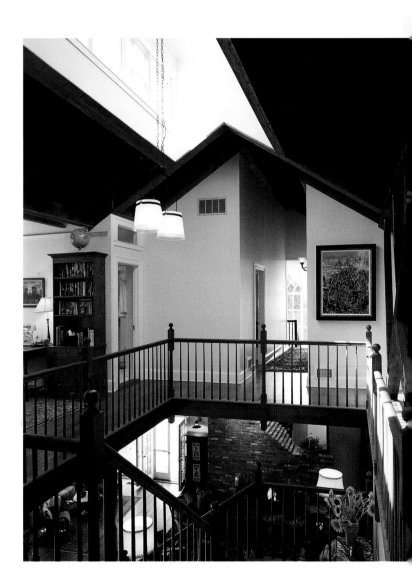

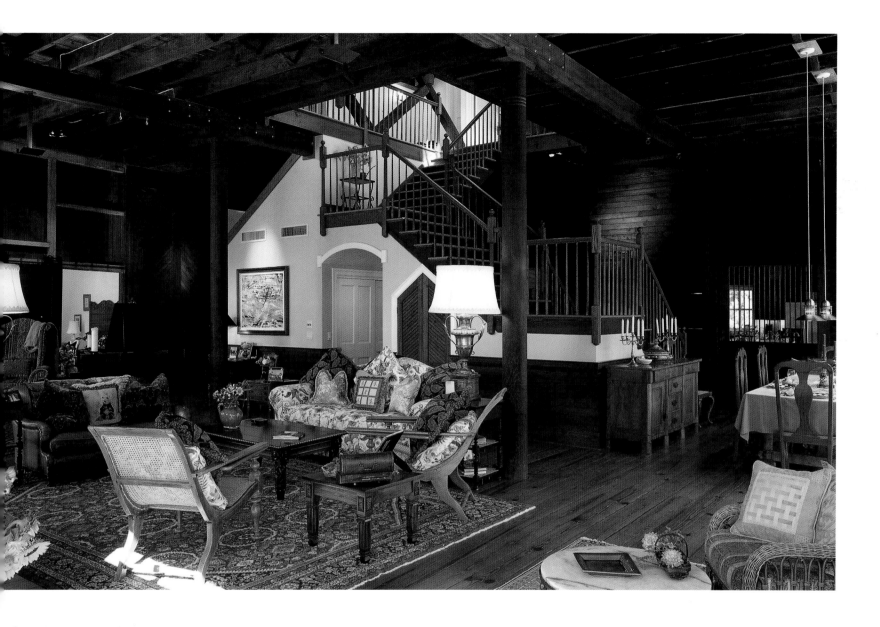

plays." The landing's popularity is enhanced by the clerestory above. Natural light spills into the center of the house, which was previously too dark to photograph.

One of the first pieces of fitness equipment installed was a swing hung from the 14-foot-high rafters in the living area. It was necessitated by an unusually wet summer, so the parents could swing the kids—then toddlers—inside. "For this beach family, during a rainy summer, it was heaven," said Coblin.

In 1993, work began on the entry and south pergola. This was the architectural extension of opening the inside out and bringing the outside in. The focus began to move into the yard with the addition of a pool, the gardens, and a driveway with the basketball hoop. Beginning with the swing/climbing equipment, the family has since put in a baseball diamond, a croquet course, a golf net, a volleyball/badminton court, a quiet swing, and a vegetable garden.

"The Carriage House is a high fit home that can change over time, that is flexible, that is organized, that makes fitness playful," said Coblin.

ABOVE: A clerestory brightens the stairs and highlights their architectural importance. Tucked away inside the stairs is storage for tennis rackets, surfboards, and bogey boards. RIGHT: Although warm and comforting, the house seems to commune with the outdoors. It's as if eating breakfast together might provoke the question, "Volleyball, anyone?"

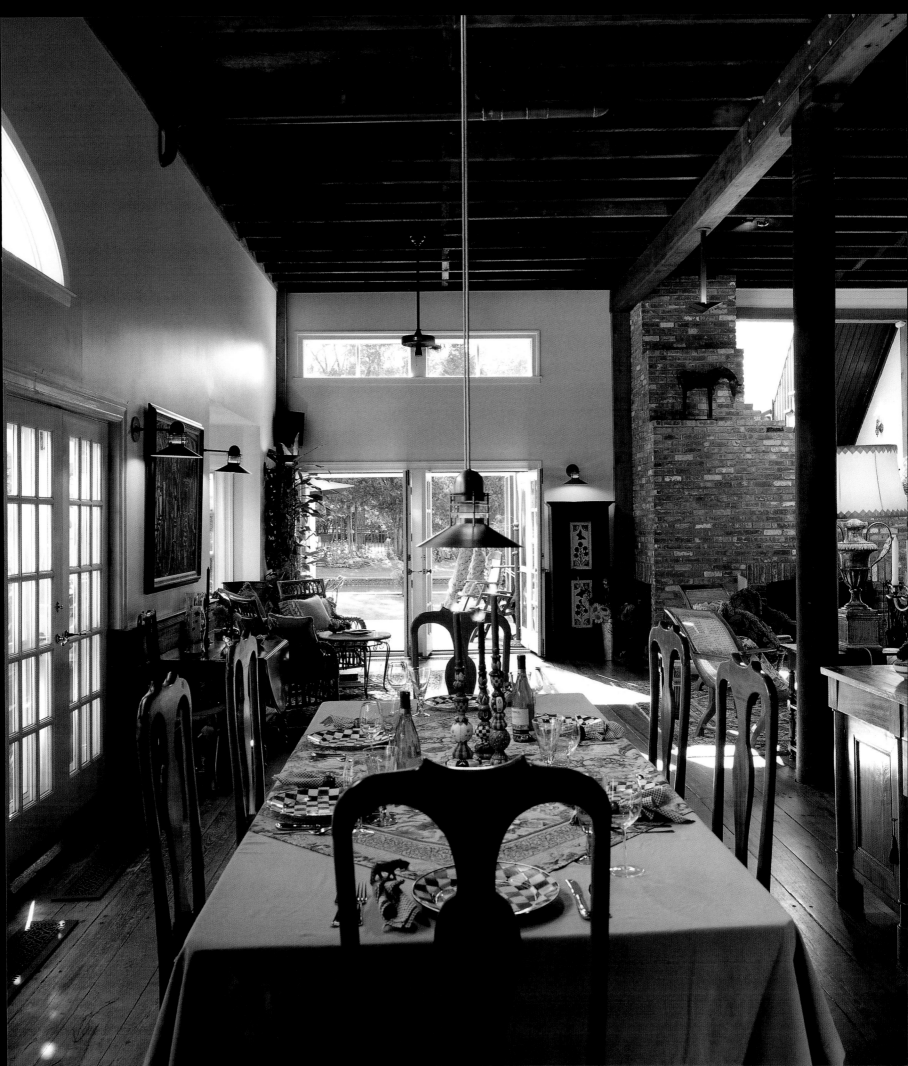

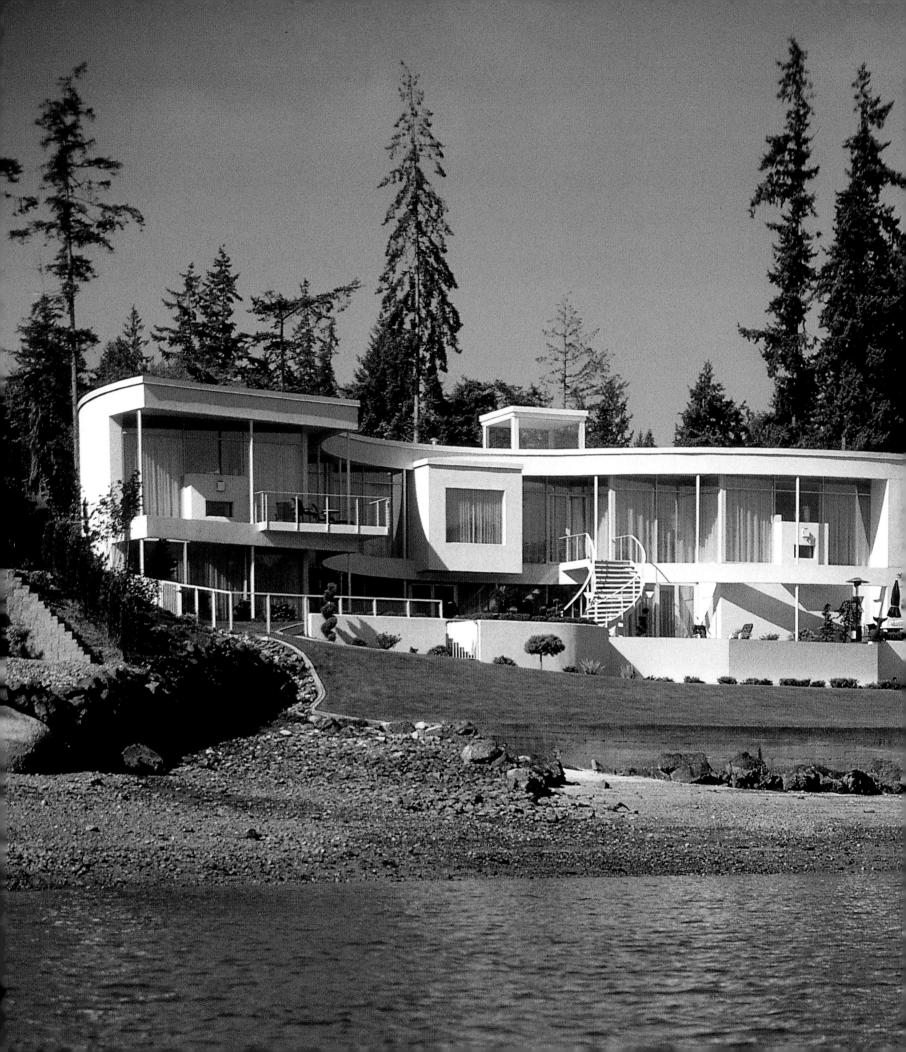

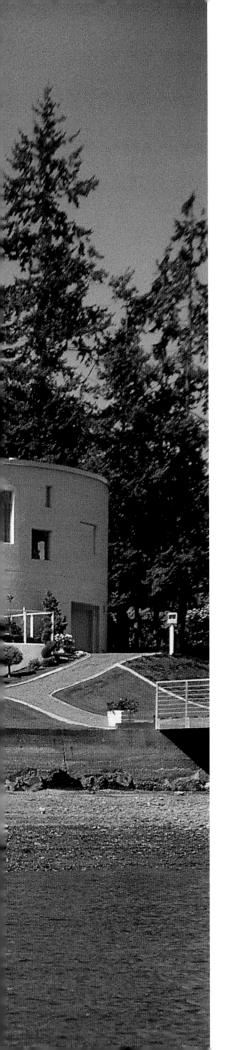

The Shape of Fitness to Come

THE ESS HOUSE

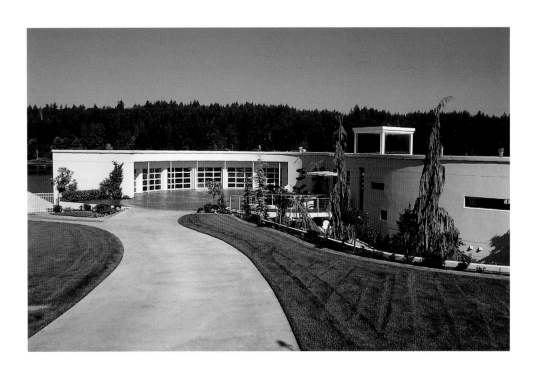

LEFT: The lower level of this Puget Sound home houses an exercise room/massage area, a separate ballet/dance studio, and a steam room, all structurally wrapped around the pool in the courtyard. **ABOVE:** The theme of fitness even influenced the design of this home. It's lines seem fluid, almost mobile.

THE TEAM OF Anderson Anderson Architecture has designed a home that serves the goal of furthering the fitness of their owners. The "Ess" House, so called for its curling shape, devotes a significant amount of space to fitness.

The Ess house is truly a high fit home, expressing the importance of fitness in its very shape, its orientation, and its space allocation. The home's "S" shape suggests movement. The snaking symmetry evolved primarily to provide privacy in the outdoor terrace area and pool, shielding it from the neighbors. The curve encircles the lower part of the house, orienting it toward the pool. The

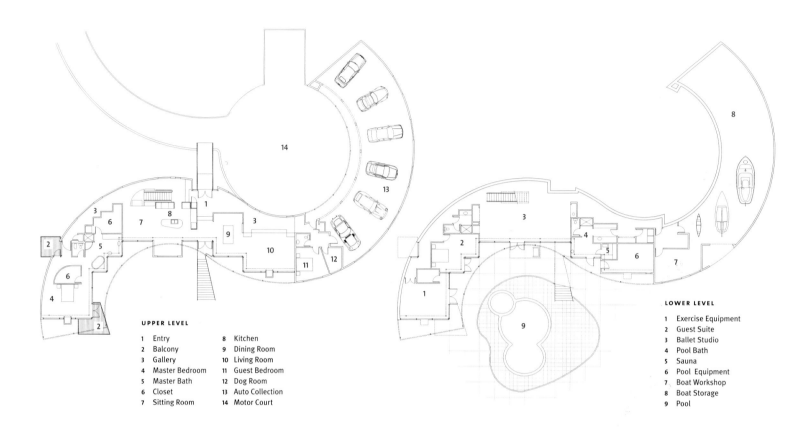

UPPER LEVEL

1	Entry	8	Kitchen
2	Balcony	9	Dining Room
3	Gallery	10	Living Room
4	Master Bedroom	11	Guest Bedroom
5	Master Bath	12	Dog Room
6	Closet	13	Auto Collection
7	Sitting Room	14	Motor Court

LOWER LEVEL

1	Exercise Equipment
2	Guest Suite
3	Ballet Studio
4	Pool Bath
5	Sauna
6	Pool Equipment
7	Boat Workshop
8	Boat Storage
9	Pool

fluid, encompassing layout eases movement between indoor and outdoor spaces devoted to various physical activities. The home's spare, sleek interiors echo a trim esthetic.

"It's a home dedicated to fitness one way or another," said Peter Anderson. "The owners take staying in shape pretty seriously."

Mostly the upper level is oriented to capture the best views of nearby Puget Sound. The lower level opens onto and encircles the pool and hot tub, with views of the sound beyond. The entire lower level of the 6,000-square-foot home is outfitted much like a well-appointed gym. The lower level also

houses an exercise room/massage area, a separate ballet/dance studio, and a steam room. A dock on the sound, just a step off the pool, moors different boats that the homeowners employ in a variety of water sports.

The home's largely prefabricated structural system allows for airy, open spaces and wide expanses of windows. Its interior reflects the owners' interest in the sleek lines of cars. It's light and trim with highly polished surfaces, acrylic, glass, lots of mirrors and high-gloss painted finishes. "The owners had auto technicians do the painting," said Anderson. "The paint they used is stronger than enamel."

RIGHT: The curvilinear shape of the home was conceived partly to provide privacy while the homeowners enjoy their swimming pool and watch sunsets on the sound. FAR RIGHT: After enjoying Puget Sound views while working out in the exercise room or ballet studio, the owners of the Ess House can swim some refreshing laps in the pool. Since the active homeowners enjoy boating, different boats are moored just a step off the pool. The home's design also factors in space for a boat workshop and boat storage.

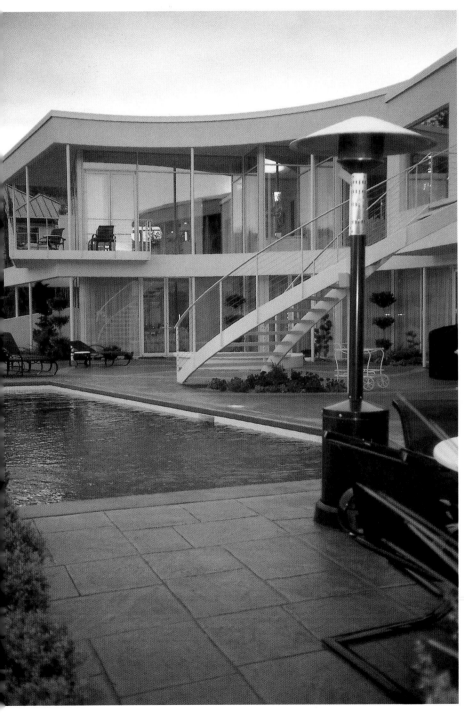

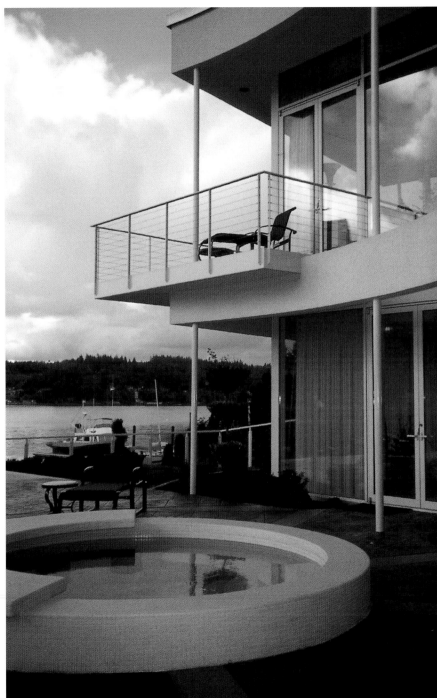

The Home as Stair Master

THE LAKE MICHIGAN HOUSE

WHEN PETER ANDERSON WAS working out the specifics of the Lake Michigan House, he asked the owners if they wanted an elevator. They declined because "running up and down stairs is good for you." Altogether, there are ten levels to the house, if you include the landing and rooftop deck, and they wanted to make full use of each flight of stairs. "It's set up so you get lots of exercise," said Anderson. "It's a StairMaster house."

Besides being an integral element of the design, visually linking all the levels, the stairs in this house are appealing in their own right. Sparely elegant, they are fashioned from semi-transparent folded steel mesh.

Each level of the house is a room, layered on top of the next, not unlike a railroad flat standing on its edge. Only one level has two rooms, the two bedrooms that the family's three children share. Otherwise there's a kitchen on one level, a living room on another, and so forth. There are no linking hallways.

All about movement, the house was designed for an active family that wanted a place where the kids could get out in the country and run around. Its towering shape is reminiscent of a high-end jungle gym structure. The surrounding land was bermed to create

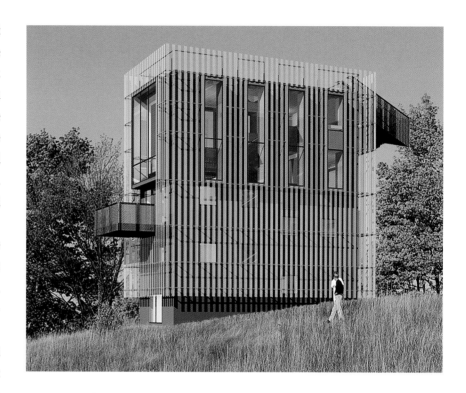

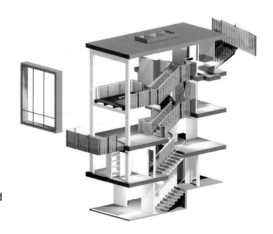

ABOVE and RIGHT: With ten levels and no elevator, this home is set up to consciously maximize the steps of a very active family. All the hallways are vertical, since stairs—rather than hallways—serve as the connecting links between rooms. Whimsical and reflective, the Lake Michigan House resembles something you might be tempted to climb in a playground.

outdoor play areas for a fort and a fire pit, and the subtle reshuffling of earth provides a gentle contrast to the tower's vertical line.

With its singular vertical presence rising above an orchard, the tower is intended to reflect the austere simplicity of the occasional farm buildings also found on the surrounding hills. The building is wrapped in a skirting wall of recycled translucent polyethylene slats, standing two feet out from the galvanized sheet-metal cladding of the wall surface. The slats are placed on aluminum frames that serve as window-washing platforms and emergency exit structures. When they are not climbing the orchard's trees, the kids might want to climb these frames. "The parents seem pretty fearless about this," said Anderson.

If the children do scale the house, it may still look like they are climbing trees. The translucent polyethylene siding material was chosen for its ability to gather the light and color of its landscape, dissolving the finely shadowed and inexplicably haloed structure into the seasonal color cycle of snow and ice and black-twig tracery, pale pink blossom clouds, pollen green, leaf and grass, and vivid foliage.

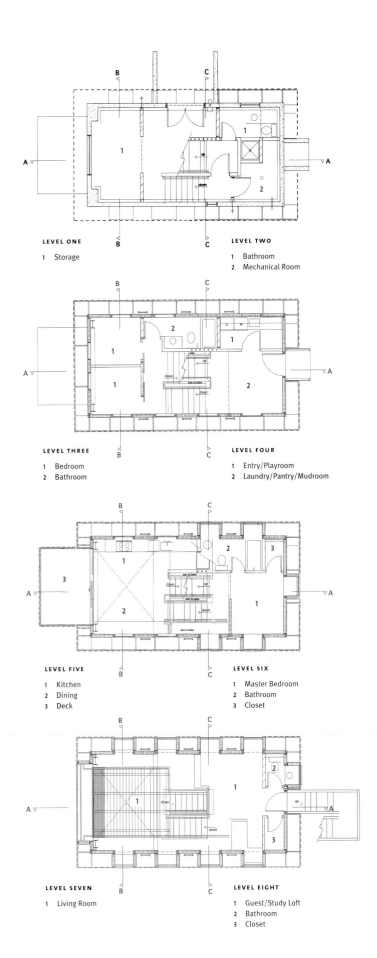

LEVEL ONE

1 Storage

LEVEL TWO

1 Bathroom
2 Mechanical Room

LEVEL THREE

1 Bedroom
2 Bathroom

LEVEL FOUR

1 Entry/Playroom
2 Laundry/Pantry/Mudroom

LEVEL FIVE

1 Kitchen
2 Dining
3 Deck

LEVEL SIX

1 Master Bedroom
2 Bathroom
3 Closet

LEVEL SEVEN

1 Living Room

LEVEL EIGHT

1 Guest/Study Loft
2 Bathroom
3 Closet

Renovating with 21st-century Priorities

THE TEN BROECK HOUSE

TWO QUESTIONS ARE GENERALLY asked when bringing a historic home into the 21st century: What's worth keeping? What's best replaced?

To add a gym, sauna, and steam room, plus a kitchen, pantry, and guest room to a neglected 18th-century homestead in Columbia County, New York, the architects Brian Messana and Toby O'Rorke first had to strip away the distractions of several earlier renovations.

"The earliest recorded date for the house is 1734, although many years of use and renovation have made the actual date unclear," said Messana. "Fabricated in hand-hewn timbers, the basic frame and form of this house conforms to frames consistent with houses built by Dutch settlers of that time."

The answer to their first question—what to get rid of—was "everything but the basic post and beam structure." The Spartan living conditions of the early settlers and the simple, clean lines of their building inspired the architects to adopt a minimal design solution. Various additions were stripped away and interior partitions removed to reveal a classic house form: "four windows, a door, and a sloped roof with a chimney on top." Inside, the rooms were reconfigured to create wider, simpler, brighter spaces.

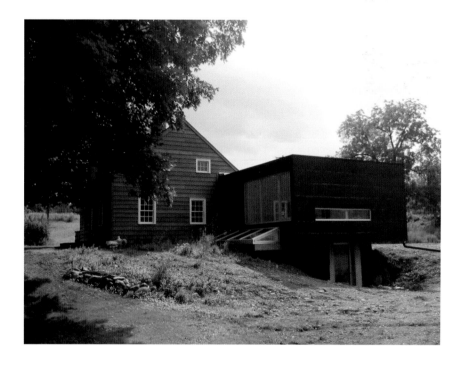

It might have been easier to knock the whole house down and start all over again, but the team tried to save what they could and build from there, preserving the spirit of the original structure. "There was history in the basement—it looks like an archeological site," said Messana. "Beautifully laid stone, beams 12 inches wide by 18 inches deep, hand-honed original pine floors, 24 inches wide. We took it apart so you could see the structural connections and modernized it."

ABOVE and **LEFT:** Looking for an unobtrusive addition to an 18th-century homestead? Why not consider a mobile home? Both have spare, simple lines. The rectangular shape of a mobile home was just what inspired an addition that expands basic living space and also houses a gym, a sauna, and a steam room. As incongruous as that might sound, the as-yet-to-be landscaped combination has a natural integrity.

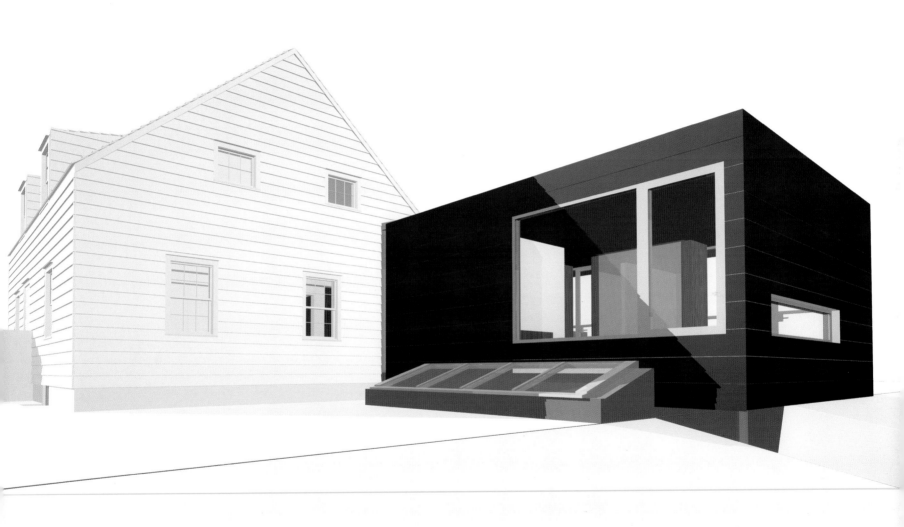

The walls were rebuilt of hand-rubbed plaster, the cedar siding replaced and all the windows re-created. A central fireplace was added to divide and define living and dining-room spaces. The only surviving finishes were some wide-board flooring and a miraculously preserved wattle and daub wall in the fieldstone basement.

After the original structure was pared down and reconfigured, that left the second question: What to add? An additional structure was needed to house a kitchen and workout space, but no solution seemed right. Rather than create a wing that would at best look patched on, Messana and O'Rorke decided to create a separate but complementary structure.

The inspiration for the new structure, which almost doubles the living space, came from vernacular mobile homes. Something about their simple rectilinear form seemed compelling and in the same spirit as the original Spartan homestead. So, the architects created a prefab addition, which is set in the footprint of the lean-to but separated from the house by a continuous 12-inch glass gasket. "The separation or gap strengthens both structures," said Messana. Instead of windows, the addition has glass panes and exterior walls clad in Cor-Ten steel, designed to rust to a point where it complements the cedar siding of the house. Besides turning to a warm brown, the rust seals and protects the structure.

The addition can be entered from the original house or from a basement door. You can walk from the dining/living room into the addition's first floor, which houses the kitchen,

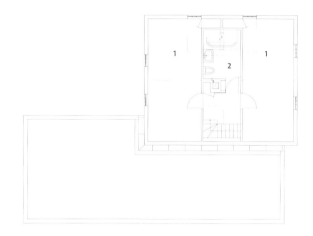

SECOND FLOOR

1 Bedroom
2 Bathroom

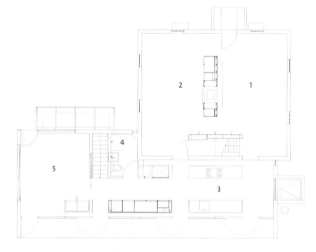

GROUND FLOOR

1 Living Room
2 Dining Room
3 Kitchen
4 Bathroom
5 Bedroom

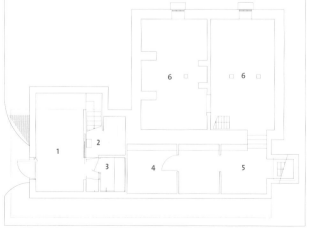

BASEMENT FLOOR

1 Exercise Room
2 Sauna
3 Steam Room
4 Storage
5 Mechanical
6 Basement

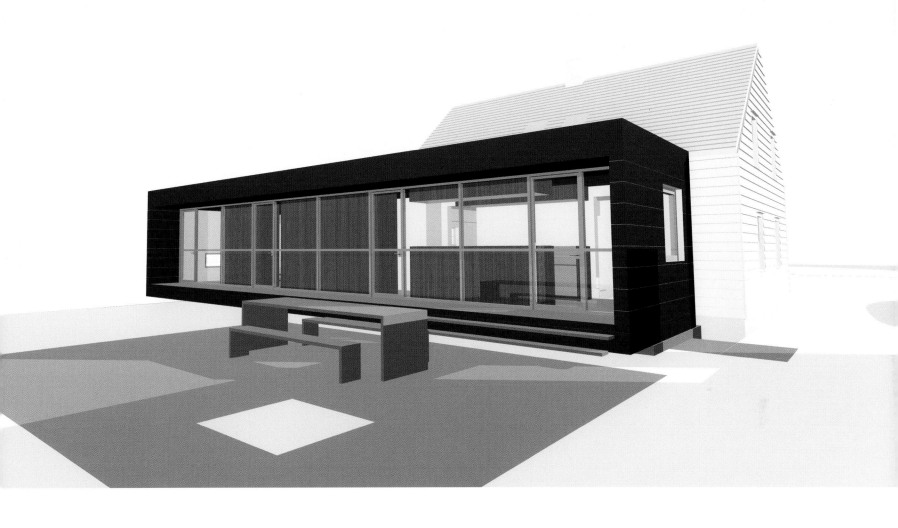

ABOVE: The prefab addition is set in the footprint of the lean-to but separated from the house by a 12-inch glass gasket. After exercise and a sauna in the lower level of the contemporary addition, opening a lower-level door will leave you facing a centuries-old apple orchard.

guest bedroom, and shower room, and then take the stairs down to the basement. Or you can walk into the basement—with the exercise, sauna, and steam rooms—from the outside. Land was excavated and regraded around the addition so that the basement was really on a "ground level." It has an outside door and plenty of windows to let in light.

To let in the maximum natural light, the gym has a skylight facing north. Its large glass door faces the four acres of apple orchards on the home's property. The steam room has sliding Plexiglas doors to let in light, and the sauna has a glass door and windows.

The gym has a flat-screen television, weights, an exercise bike, and a treadmill. Here, the Portuguese limestone floor, shared by the sauna and steam room, is covered by a rubber mat for sit-ups. Radiant heating keeps floors and toes warm in the colder seasons. There's a stereo system and mirrors, plus the seasonally changing view of the apple orchards, probably similar to that enjoyed by the homestead's original Dutch settlers.

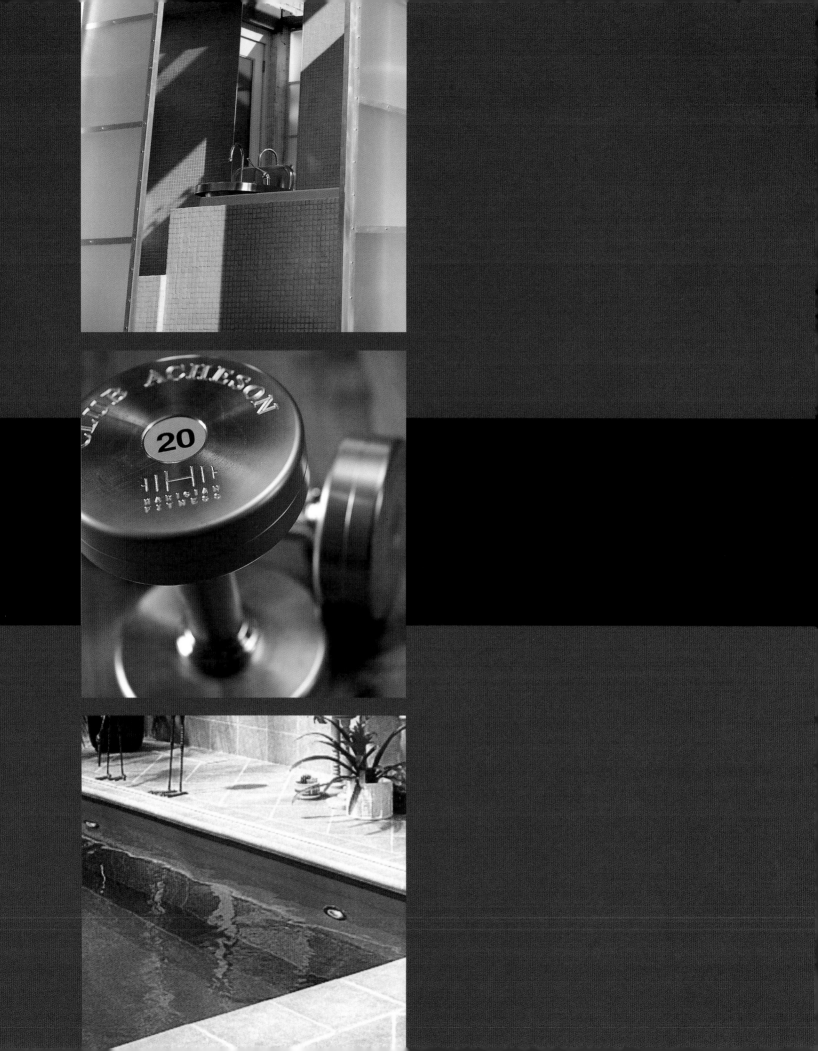

elements

The Active Design

THERE IS NOTHING NEW about some of the elements used in the high fit home—only a newfound appreciation for their ability to shift the human shape. For centuries there have been homes where layouts encouraged extra steps, often much to their owners' chagrin. Houses have been built around exercise space as far back as the Roman atrium. Some homes have more than their fair share of stairs, others have vantage points that promote stair climbing.

Le Corbusier's Villa Savoie in Poissy, France, with its terrace roof garden, might be considered an example of the latter. Climbing up to a garden consumes more calories than walking out a door. Visiting the roof garden seems like the culmination of the home's design.

As Le Corbusier once said of a project, the "house will be rather like an architectural promenade. You enter: the architectural spectacle at once offers itself to the eye. You follow an itinerary and the perspectives develop with great variety, developing a play of light on the walls or making pools of shadow. Large windows open up views of the exterior where the architectural unity is reasserted. Here, reborn for our modern eye, are historic architectural discoveries: the pilotis, the long windows, the roof garden, the glass facade. Once again we must learn at the end of the day to appreciate what is available."

What is available in the high fit home are the basics—internal and external layout, stairs and specific spaces. All of these can conspire to improve us.

Layout

There are many ways the floor plan of a house can multiply the number of steps taken in the course of daily life. A snaking design or sequential, "railroad-flat" design (whether built horizontally or vertically) necessitates extra steps to get to different rooms.

A camp-style layout conjures up opportunities to amble from unit to unit and discover new perspectives. Separate second-floor units that are not connected but must be approached by their own set of stairs may not necessarily make daily chores easier but they can certainly make the people who live there more muscular. Home plans that devote a significant percentage of floor space to exercise place a high value on it, while a home with a gym near the front door or near the kitchen makes working out a daily priority.

In one home designed by Abramson Teiger, the gym is placed conveniently next to the kitchen. This makes it easier to reach during the day—but the placement could also help keep excess snacking in check. If you could see the stationary bike on which you would have to spend an hour to burn off the calories from those cookies, would you eat them?

RIGHT: Placing exercise equipment or workout rooms in a visible or highly trafficked location can remind you of the importance of working out. Why not place your gym near the front door or near the kitchen? Or perhaps the whole family might benefit from a family room/gym?

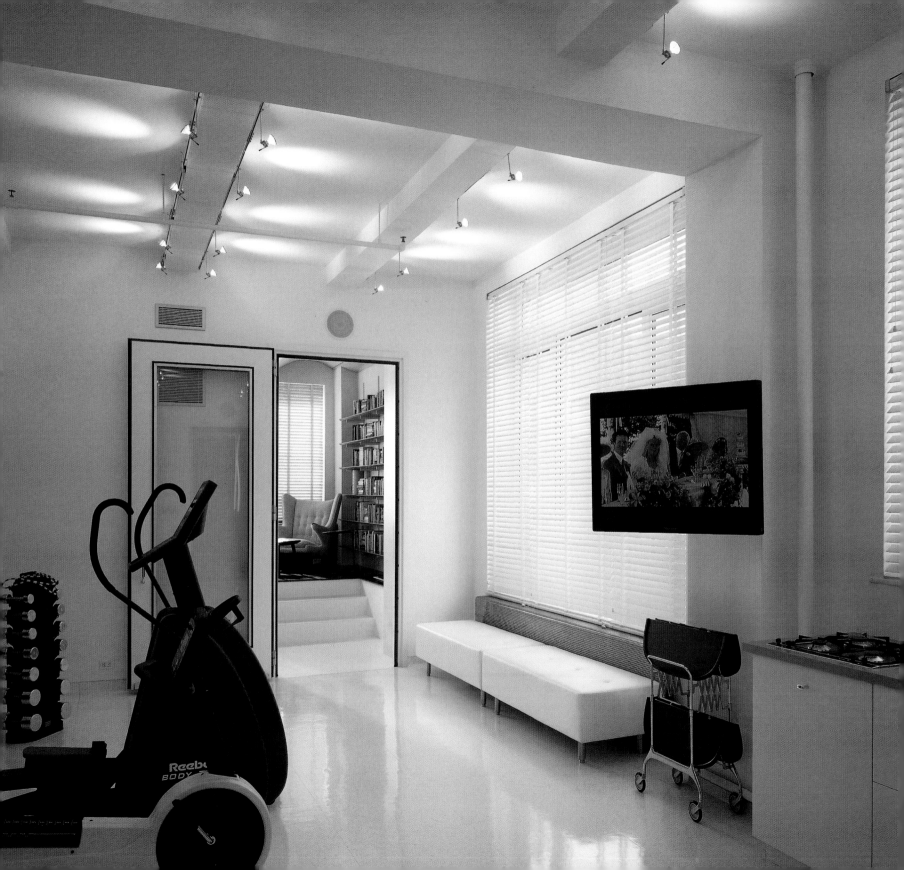

Stairs and Ramps

Stairs are one architectural feature that can be good for your health. Walking up stairs is great exercise for the heart, legs, and lungs. A half-hour of climbing steep stairs at home can burn up to 300 calories. While few people climb stairs for half an hour at a stretch, the trips up and down stairs during the course of a day can add up. Think that's not enough justification to add a flight of stairs?

A recent British study found that women walking continuously for 30 minutes five days a week had almost identical increases in fitness as women who split their 30 minutes into three 10-minute walks. The brief walkers also lost more weight. Every flight of stairs counts and should be an essential part of the equation.

Architects have a new rationale to add stairs at the planning stage, as did Anderson Anderson in their Lake Michigan House, or to envision stair construction that invites climbing. Well-thought-out stairs become a living space in their own right when their vertical unfurling includes somewhere to display collections, a place to perform home-grown children's productions, or a cozy place to read. Upward odysseys are all the more likely if stairs or ramps are more spacious and attractive or have one or more enticing vantage points, as in the Spine House designed by Sir Nicholas Grimshaw with Mark Bryden and Martin Wood.

New takes on the home have made it more practical to add a flight of stairs or, for that matter, the room to which the stairs will lead. Prefab homes that can arrive as a single unit may also have the option of adding another room later. Consider the case of the "up! house" designed by Craig Konyk, which gives homeowners a chance to step up to a fitness floor at any time. The beauty of the up! house is its elasticity, its ability to ensure future flexibility.

Add a Gym Whenever!

Perhaps there's no time, need, or budget for exercise space now, but in a few years, shifting goals or shapes could make it a priority. An increasingly popular idea for a first-time homeowner is the prefab with room for quick and easy growth. The dynamic up! house is elevated off the ground, which already necessitates increased use of stairs, but a prefab also includes the potential for additional rooms, one of which can be a gym, customized to the owner's requirements.

"It's kind of like a house doing calisthenics," said Konyk. "It's not just a house sitting on the ground, it's kind of a youthful energetic idea for a house."

The up! house starts with a two-bedroom 1,500-square-foot model that can be customized to grow upward. Built with superinsulating, highly recyclable polyisoprene metal exterior panels, the durable steel-frame construction is available in 14 factory-applied automotive colors. The highly resistant exterior paint is stronger than enamel. Flush-insulated operable windows feature mouse-gray tinted glass, often used in car exterior windows, for maximum daytime privacy. Minimum site foundations save on-site labor costs and free up valuable yard area for parking and outdoor fitness.

RIGHT: No room for a gym? No problem. This energetic prefab home offers opportunities to add rooms—including gyms—as needed. The dynamic up house seems poised to jump up off of its foundation.

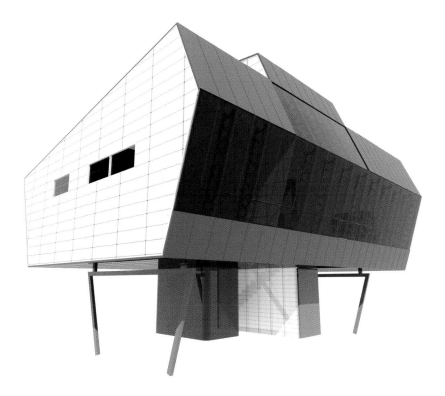

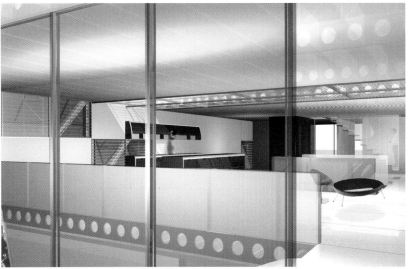

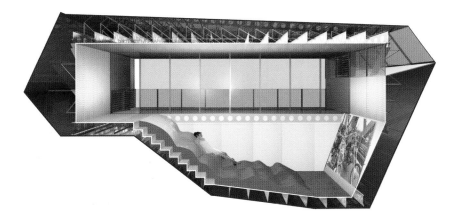

Home as a Fitness Center

A home can also be a family's own health club. With or without such movement-inducing features as elongated layouts or additional staircases, homes can optimize health by offering the tools, space, and access for indoor and outdoor activities. Indoor activity spaces can include gyms, pools, basketball courts, squash courts, dance studios, yoga or Pilates spaces, spas, and saunas. Fitness can create a place where the family meets to play.

Outdoor activities can be fostered by plotting a home design around a yard or a pool, or by facilitating access to such outdoor fun as hiking, boating, or swimming.

Or a high fit home can be a getaway such as a ski lodge or beach house—the vacation choice for those who relax by revving up their metabolism.

At-Home Spas

The at-home spa is one of the latest trends in bath design, offering a personal space for pampering and a way to soothe aching muscles after a workout. A home spa can be part of a bathroom. It can also be included in a larger exercise area, or it can be the hub of a room that includes a small exercise area, such as a space for yoga or meditation. Ideally, a spa room is designed to be serene and have multiple sources of mood-restoring light.

Adding a skylight or dividing the spa room with glass walls or blocks can maximize natural light. Desirable features may include a steam shower, a soaking tub, and floors warmed by radiant heating.

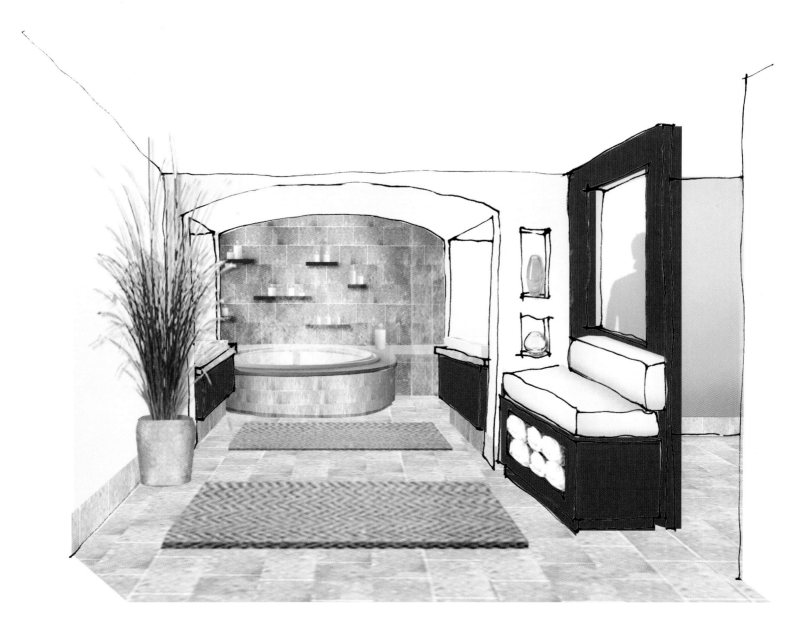

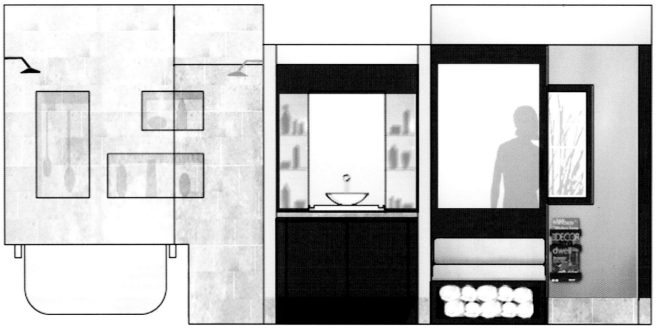

One serene example of a spa that soothes and promotes family togetherness is the bathroom spa, built by the architect-designer Michelle Kaufman and her colleague Camille Urban Jobe. The Chun Spa was built as a project for an HGTV design show, selected from one of three proposed designs. The couple who selected their work rarely has any time together, so having a beautiful environment to relax in after a workout is a priority. To accomplish this, Kaufman and Urban Jobe transformed their bathroom into a spa retreat.

The room, located next to the couple's exercise space, is divided into three zones, with the front zone for lounging, reading, and hanging out. The center space has an archway with two sinks embedded into opposite sides of the arch, so that when husband and wife perform morning ablutions, they can see each other's reflections. The back space has what Kaufman calls a "firewall" of dark, rich red stone. That space contains a hidden toilet and a walk-in shower with a steamer.

When the steamer goes off, the red stone becomes a richer, darker color. On the firewall are many shelves lined with candles to illuminate the room when there's no natural light. A whirlpool tub has water pouring from a ceiling spout, expressly designed for its soothing sound.

"We were trying to take basic elements such as fire, water, air, and earth and really accentuate them in the space," said Kaufman. "For more of the water element, we used a sink where the water runs over a flat slab, so there's no bowl, kind of like an infinity pool."

There was little natural light to work with, since the section of the house was embedded in a hill. The team brightened the space by using a lot of glass and natural stone. Wood trim in an espresso color sets off the tile and serves as a stabilizing contrast. Besides making it a healthier, visually cleaner space, the renovation also adds enough room for a massage table the couple can use for a reviving massage at home.

"As many people have brought the office home, they are also bringing athleticism home," said Kaufman. "They are finding a way to take better care of their bodies at home."

A Spa Grows in Brooklyn

Although Brooklyn is a bustling part of New York City, it's a borough with many tree-lined streets and plenty of green space for exercise and the occasional personal retreat.

Creating a healing oasis of calm in an urban setting was the idea behind this spa addition to a circa 1885 Park Slope townhouse. The brownstone owners asked the architects Murdock Young to replace a small existing backyard greenhouse with a sunny, multipurpose living space for year-round use—a space that would bring the house into the garden and the garden into the house. Their approach was to design a flexible indoor-outdoor space that maximized sunlight and a direct connection to the outdoor garden while maintaining the option of privacy.

Since having a place to revive your spirits is an important part of staying mentally and physically healthy in a stressful city environment, the homeowners built the addition before renovating the home's interior.

ABOVE LEFT: A "firewall" of rich red stone is illuminated by candles in this home spa retreat, designed for post-workout use. When a steamer goes off, the steam seems to deepen and enrich the wall's color. BELOW LEFT: The center part of the spa has an archway with two embedded sinks, one on each side, to allow simultaneous use to facilitate morning conversations.

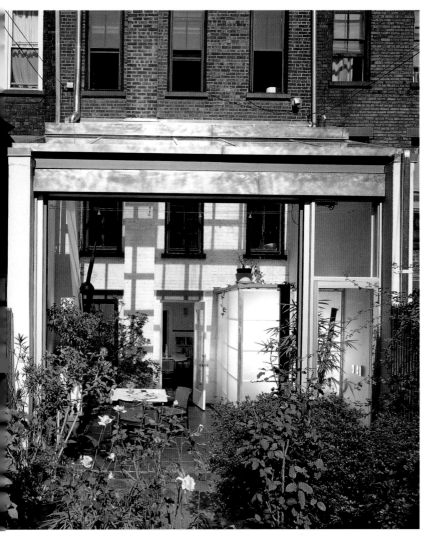
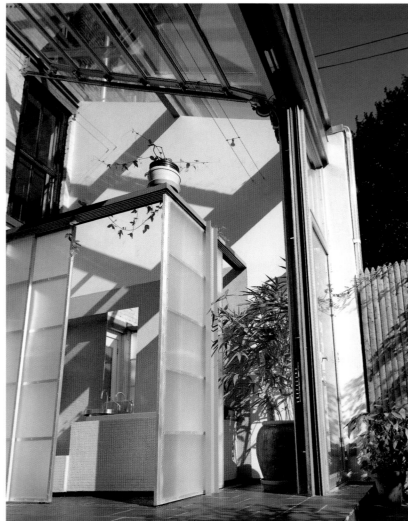

"The space is all about relaxing," said Shea Murdock. Since the homeowner and Murdock are both cyclists, they had an easy rapport on exactly what would be soothing after coming home from a long bike ride.

The extension is bathed in light during the day and glows from within after dark. To maximize the influx of daylight, the double-height space of glass, concrete, and steel is adorned with a glass roof and features an oversized glass garage door. A second enclosure inside defines an area for the sink and tub. Sliding aluminum and fiberglass panels, inspired by Japanese shoji screens, allow the space to be opened up to the room and garden or closed off for privacy. At night, the back-lit enclosure illuminates the living space, creating a beacon of light. "Successive levels of transparency succeed in connecting the inside to the outside and bringing the garden into the space," said Shea.

To connect the indoors to the outdoors visually, patterned pavers of slate extend the flooring into the garden. The extension is connected to the kitchen on the ground floor, providing a place to eat on nice evenings. In the summer, an operable skylight lets air circulate in. On chilly nights, a gas-burning fireplace makes it more atmospheric.

ABOVE LEFT: This double-height space of glass and concrete serves as a retreat from city cares. Having a glass roof, it is filled with natural light during the day. At night, the room seems to glow from within. **ABOVE RIGHT:** Layers of transparent material veil the spa from prying eyes. **RIGHT:** Pavers of slate extend the flooring of the spa into the garden. Beyond the lush backyard oasis, towers a line of Brooklyn brownstones.

high fit home

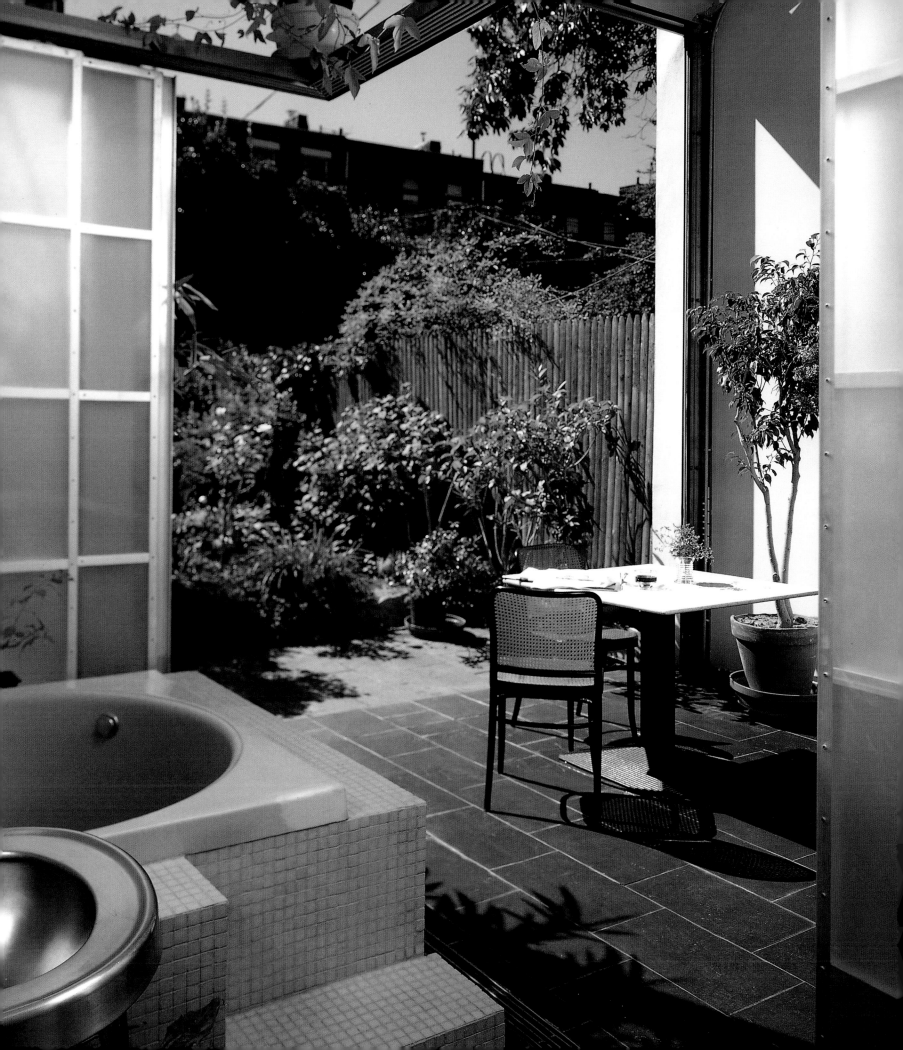

Gyms

PERHAPS THE MOST popular workout space being added to homes today is the gym. A sleek elliptical machine tucked into the corner of the master bedroom or weights resting on a home-office filing cabinet may be as ambitious as some people get, but increasingly the home gym is seen as a distinct and necessary space, with its own highly specialized furnishings and ornamentation. If the rest of your home has character and individual style, says this new design sensibility, why should that space be any less than expressive of your taste?

In one man's combination study/workout area fashioned for a showcase house by the California designer Cheryl Gardner, a few minutes of writer's block can be alleviated by a few minutes on the treadmill.

"Rather than a separate gym, they wanted a man's retreat," said Gardner of the project, which she worked on with the architect Richard Landry.

The fitness equipment she chose was a high-end treadmill with a built-in 15-inch plasma-screen TV and some dumbbells. Rather than partition a section of the room for exercise equipment, Gardner chose to treat the treadmill as a piece of furniture and balance its presence. The treadmill is almost exactly the same dimensions as the 1940s desk—six feet long by 30 inches wide—and was treated with the same compositional respect.

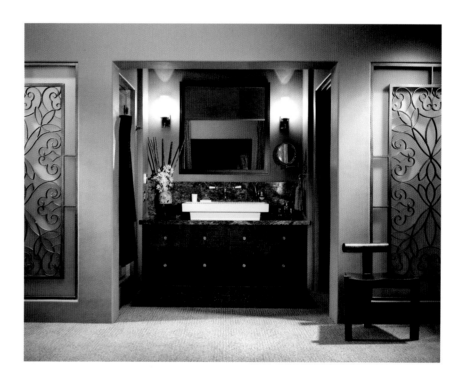

"The house was Andalusian, the equipment was modern, so I introduced elements from different periods. Balanced correctly, it all works," said Gardner. "Balanced, it becomes art."

With its splashes of clear reds and blues, the black lines of the modern equipment and the stylized postwar furniture, the room does indeed have the eclectic feel of a Kandinsky painting. The oval racetrack shape of the treadmill's base is echoed in the oval shape of the 1940s desk, with its shiny nickel accents. The chrome legs of the blue, patent-leather bench, separating the treadmill and desk, mirror the chrome of the dumbbells.

ABOVE: This man's study/ workout area designed for a California showcase house places fluid Andalusian design elements within rectangular architectural forms, creating a feeling of movement within a confined space. RIGHT: In this room, the treadmill has become an essential piece of furniture, echoing forms and colors found throughout the room.

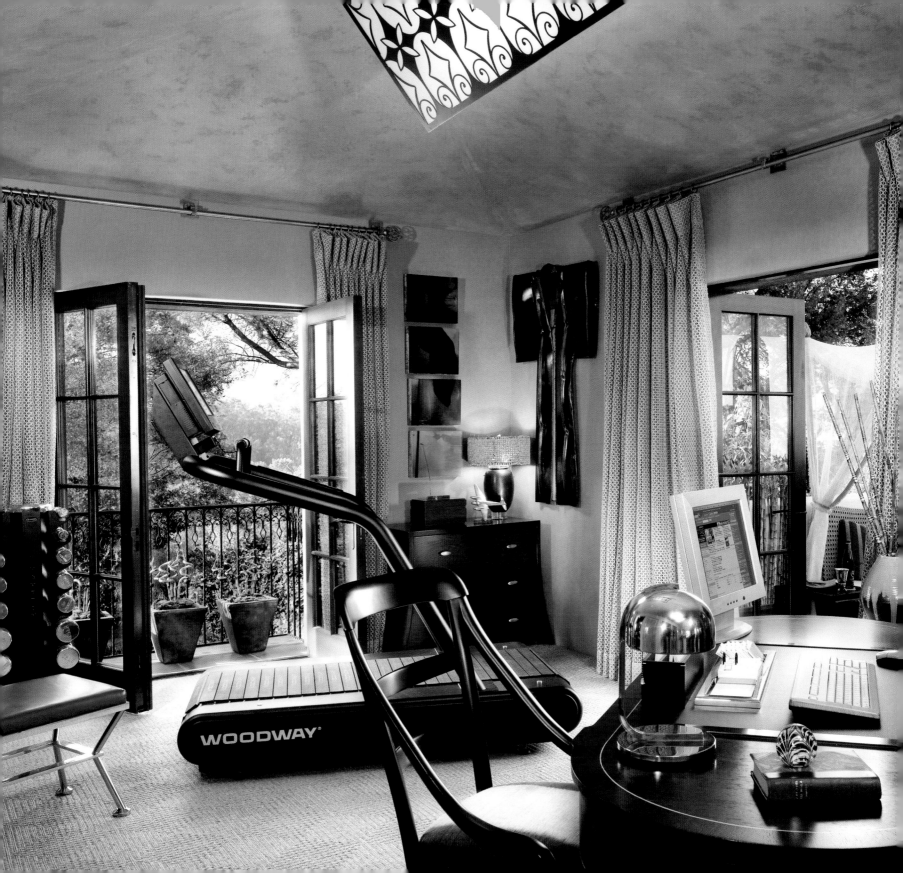

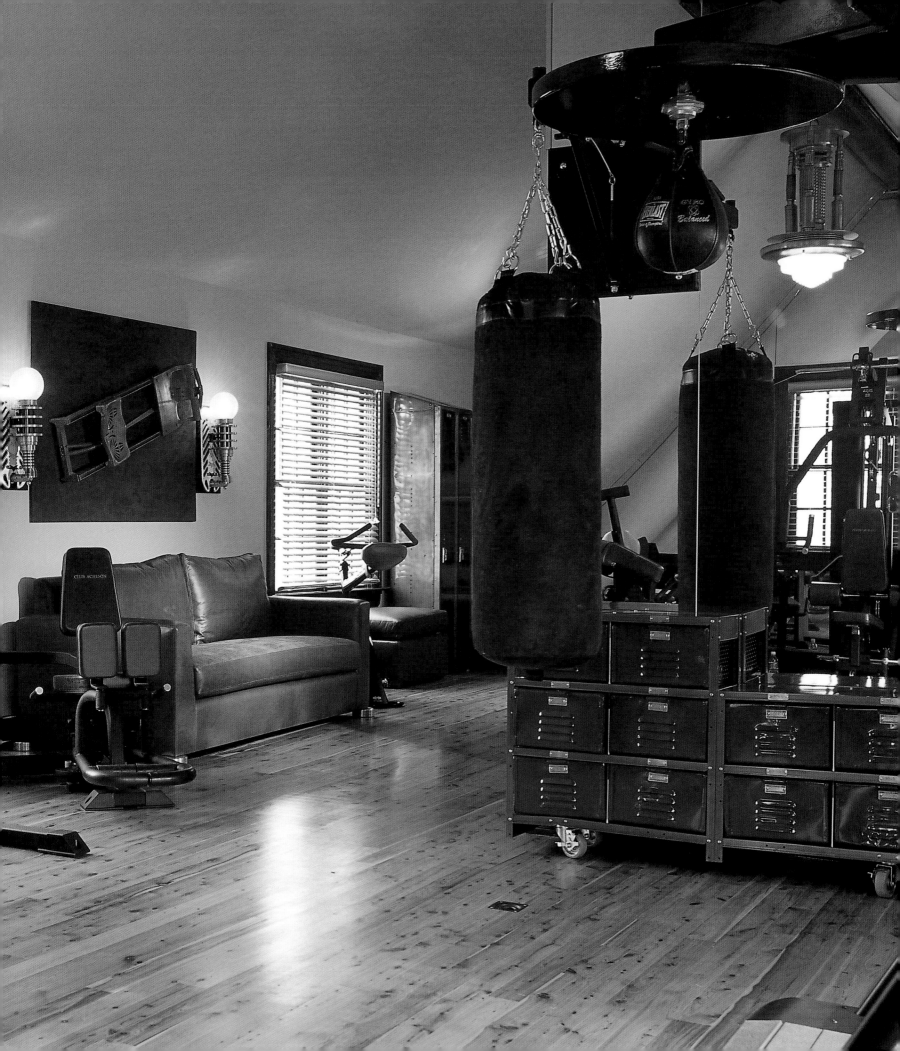

Gardner created a custom chandelier of laser-cut steel and antique bronze and added a stainless steel water cooler for post exercise replenishment. Mirrors amplify the room's many metallic accents and make it seem even bigger and more open; patio doors provide ventilation. The floors are carpeted with abaca, used throughout the house. Gardner's treatment put the exercise equipment in perspective, so it would not "take over" the room.

If space is an issue, a workout space can double as a guest room as it did in Joel Sanders's Millennium Loft. Or a homeowner may also choose to renovate an existing space, such as the basement or garage. Gyms and small pools can fit into some basements, if there's enough light and the ceilings are high enough. Attics are a possibility, although few are roomy and ventilated well-enough. Even barns are now being retrofitted with high-tech toning equipment.

There's always the possibility of adding a wing that either blends into the period of the home or has its own style to fit the spirit of the house. Or you can build a separate structure that becomes part of a domestic campus.

Gym Design

Although the dictates of a gym's function mean fabric and fittings are often kept to a minimum, color, materials, and lighting can still be design considerations. These decorative elements help add personality to a potentially sterile space.

According to Naomi Leff, the designer responsible for conceiving the lush, opulent interiors of Ralph Lauren's flagship stores,

"Unless it's a smaller apartment in a building with a gym, practically every home design now has some kind of gym in it. It's a challenge decorating them. In gyms, the equipment plays a powerful role in the design."

"Although putting the equipment in that room will make it look like a gym," says Leff, there is always some room for added panache.

"You can acknowledge the general ambience in the house. A house with a light feeling might have blond wood flooring and white or blond leather on the equipment," said Leff. "Also, I don't like to put lights in the ceiling because then you are looking up at the lights."

To avoid the distraction and eye fatigue effects of overhead lighting, some designers use "floating" mirrors off walls and ceilings so fixtures can be installed behind them.

"When designing the gym," cautions Leff, "remember that you will need a lot of power. Many pieces of exercise equipment plug in."

And don't forget to give it some element of your personality.

Kids' Stuff

With one in five children, aged 6 to 17, overweight, it's not just adults who need to get in gear. More parents are giving kids the gear to get in shape. The idea of children working out on gym equipment may seem odd to some but, under the right conditions, children have a lot to gain from strength training and endurance exercises.

As families strive against the alarming obesity statistics, "tweens" and teens are becoming two of the fasting-growing demographic groups served by the health and

LEFT: To make this gym feel like a place in which to have fun, master gym designer Mark Harigian added a touch of nostalgic fantasy with retro lighting and vintage Pepsi machines. In this cross between a tree house and a clubhouse, state-of-the-art steel customized exercise equipment is reflected on the warmly glowing custom flooring.

gyms

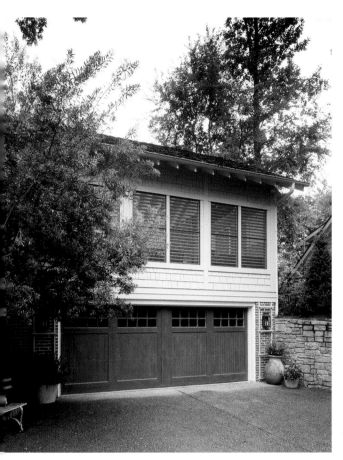

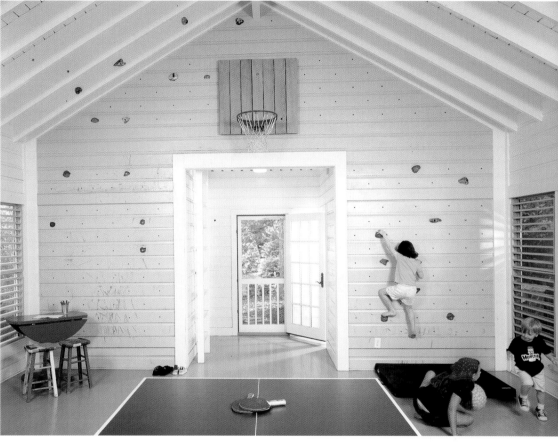

fitness industry. The number of Americans younger than 18 who belong to health clubs already exceeds four million.

The National Association for Sports and Physical Education recommends that children 6 to 11 exercise for 30 to 60 minutes a day—and that's a lot more than most kids get. The average child watches 21 hours of television every week. If parents can decrease that to only seven hours a week, they can cut a child's risk of obesity in half.

How do you divert children away from the flickering allure of the television and the instant gratification of the computer? Besides serving as a good example by exercising themselves, parents can create spaces that foster movement. Such kid-friendly modifications can range from adding the classic basketball hoop over the garage door or a jungle gym in the backyard to transforming the entire garage or basement into a kid-centric gym.

Another option is to add scaled-down exercise equipment to the home gym—sometimes with an added electronic perk to ease the transition. Some child-size treadmills and bicycles feature electronic games that children can play while emulating grown-ups. One type of interactive exercise bike spurs friendly competition by providing computer games on which children can race each other.

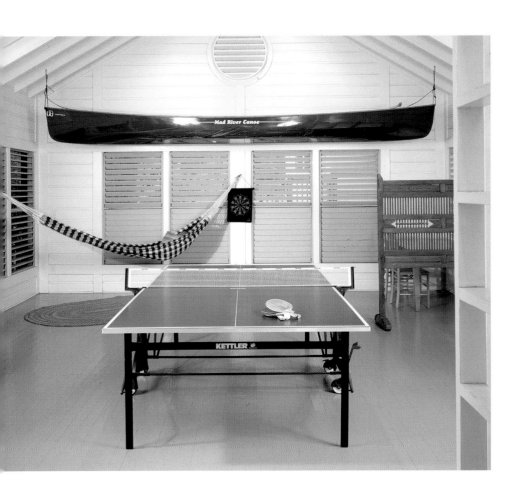

The idea was to create a neighborhood retreat, a place that seemed remote, that seemed to belong to the children, and yet remained under the watchful eye of their parents.

"It was a fun project," said Eric Rothman, design director for HammerSmith, an Atlanta-based design-build firm specializing in renovations. The firm transformed a shell of a garage—merely a foundation slab and two retaining walls—into a two-car garage on the first story, topped by a pool house, a gymnasium complete with basketball hoop, a room for table tennis, a rock-climbing wall, a guest room, a changing room, and a bathroom.

The pool, which already existed when the family moved in, is a few steps down from the garage's second level on the left. On the way in from the pool, is a shallow hip roof that looks almost flat. On the left is a full bath and on the right is a changing room. From the central hallway, a ladder climbs to a nine-foot-high "sleepover" loft space built within the roof.

The main gymnasium is a big, open space with a basketball hoop and adjustable climbing walls that provide another way to reach the sleeping loft.

The climbing wall is 9 feet on one side and goes to 16 or 17 feet on the other. Children can climb the walls to a window that lets them into the sleeping loft. The walls were designed to be as flexible as possible, accommodating growing limbs. Every 12 to 15 inches, holes are drilled into the plywood in a diamond pattern. "Rock" footholds are attached with threaded

ABOVE FAR LEFT: This farmhouse-style two-car garage in an Atlanta suburb is actually a family fitness center where children can play table tennis, basketball, climb, and swim. **ABOVE LEFT:** Children can ascend the built-in climbing wall to the sleepover loft space. **ABOVE:** The homeowners constructed this family fitness center—complete with table tennis—so that their children would have a place to hang out with friends, while remaining safely within the range of parental radar.

Rock-climbing walls are also an increasingly popular family-friendly choice. Climbing is second nature to most kids. A section of adult climbing walls can be modified for children, with shorter walls and large holds that are easier for small hands to grip.

Family Gym

The family that plays together often finds a way to fit play into their renovation plans. That was the case with one Atlanta family that wanted to transform their rudimentary garage into a playhouse—a space that would promote fitness and encourage their children's friends to hang out there.

metal pins that screw into metal-lined holes. The rocks can be repositioned to make climbing easier or more challenging.

The front walls are of wood siding. The designers used ship-lap siding and put it on the walls backward. The tongue-and-groove planks fit together tightly to create the summer camp feeling and also look like an 18th-century log cabin in the woods. The floors are painted pine, which is covered by different kinds of mats for different kinds of energy.

"In this space you literally have kids bouncing off the walls. It needs to be tough, easy to maintain, and it has character," says Rothman, who designed the space to grow with the kids and become a gym for the grown-ups when the kids move out.

A challenge faced by the firm was the pedigree of the house. Since the classic, cottage craftsman home was designed in the early 1900s by Neil Reed, a well-known Atlanta architect, and stood in the heart of a historic neighborhood, the garage would not only have to pass muster with the family that would use it but need a nod of approval from the neighbors. The project's facade would have to be classic and gracious. While the inside of the 450-square-foot gym/garage looks more like a summer camp, the outside, with its louvered windows, shutters, and farmhouse style, looks more like a cottage.

"We picked up details from the house and tied them together in what a garage of that era would have had," said Rothman. "We had to go through historic district approval and we passed with flying colors."

Climbing Walls

The climbing wall is easily the most upwardly mobile form of exercise equipment. A climbing wall can range from a few feet in height to hundreds of feet in gyms or outdoor spaces, but most home indoor climbing walls are limited to the size of the space they're in.

Most climbing walls are built indoors, since using the structure of the building helps keep costs down and allows climbing in a controlled environment. To make indoor climbing worth it, however, the walls need to be scale-worthy in height. A garage can be a good place to install a climbing wall, because many garages have large, open spaces. If your basement ceiling is high enough, a shorter wall can give you something to do while waiting for the laundry or give children a place to burn up some energy.

A linear climbing wall attached to the side of a garage or a stone basement wall can give small children the benefit of climbing without the dangers of scaling a tall wall. The handholds in such walls come in imaginative shapes (squiggles, letters, or numbers), fixed a short, safe distance from the floor so kids won't need ropes or harnesses. Some climbing walls are "dry erase," so kids can write on them. Words or numbers can also be magnetically attached to the walls to create learning games. Smaller children can climb on letters or number; older children can remove certain words from the wall as they define them or numbers as they perform equations. It's even

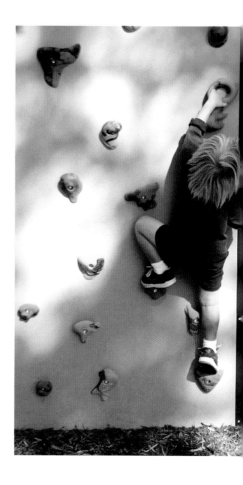

ABOVE: Climbing walls for children now have something to say. With pegs that double as letters, climbers can also learn to spell or play word games. Some come with dry erase surfaces so you can write on them. ABOVE RIGHT: A kid-size climbing wall can promote upward mobility and plenty of exercise.

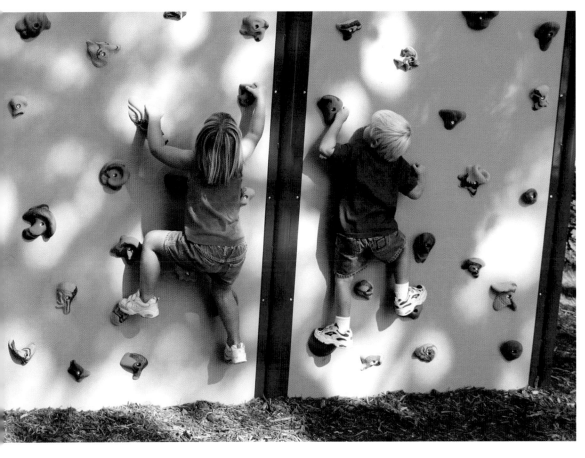 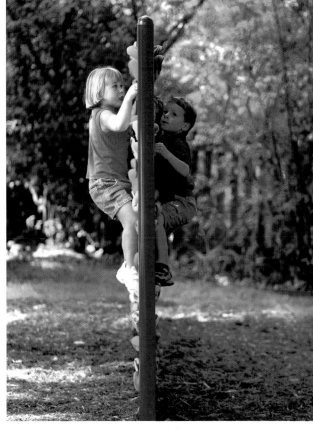

possible to play aerobic word games. A safety floor mat can soften tumbles.

Climbing walls have also given new life to the silos found on farms, since these structures already have the height necessary for an interesting climb, says Timothy Sudeith of Everlasting Climbing Walls. The firm recently added a climbing wall to a silo in a barn that was already retrofitted with a basketball court and showers.

A heightened appreciation for climbing has also prompted homeowners to erect outdoor climbing walls as a form of high-fit sculpture. Though limited by inclement weather, an outdoor climbing wall's height is not limited, unless the neighbors or local ordinances object.

Or you could import your own boulders. Depending on their dimensions, these fit-right-in-with-the-landscaping,hand-sculpted climbing structures can be fun for kids and the professional climber. Faux boulders, available in concrete, poly resin, and wood, can be fitted with handholds.

It is possible to build your own indoor climbing wall, but it's very important that you have enough structural support and that holds are securely fastened. The safest bet is to have an expert install it, or at the very least inspect your job.

Master Gym Designer

MARK HARIGIAN

ALTHOUGH SCIENTISTS CAN ONLY hypothesize about the future of home fitness technology, Mark Harigian, known as the "architect of the anatomy," has not only seen this future—he already helps create it in the homes of the rich and powerful.

Boldly venturing where no one had gone before, Harigian, the founder of Los-Angeles-based Harigian Fitness, was asked to design the gym on TV's starship *Enterprise*. A futuristic spaceship gym was not such a cosmic leap, because he already uses cutting-edge technology not only to custom-fit his clients but to heighten their motivation. The best way, he says, to get people to make the most of their equipment is by creating a personal workout environment that makes exercise exciting.

Since motivation is very individual, Harigian works to uncover just what might propel his clients. He does a personal profile, finding out what interests the person he's designing for and what makes that person's wish list.

For one movie mogul who had always wanted to climb Mount Everest but was not ready to scale the entire mountain, Harigian set up a base camp on the mountain, helicoptered in chefs to re-create a five-star environment, and arranged for manageable day treks. He made videos of the landscape that the client could view during treadmill workouts. That way the client could employ fantasy to spark a workout reality.

There are as many ways to motivate through design as there are people who want to exercise. Will a koi pond winding through your walnut floor induce you to spend more time on the treadmill? Or how about a plasma-screen TV that plays favorite running routes, coordinated so that the treadmill track inclines to simulate any steepness shown on the screen? Or how about swimming or rowing to wave images coordinated with the intensity of the current programmed into your endless pool?

A waterfall; personally engraved weight-training equipment; super flexible subflooring; retro light fixtures a la Flash Gordon; a comfy leather sofa for the clubhouse effect; a 50-gallon copper soaking tub to soothe those aching muscles. Creating rooms with these custom touches is all in a day's work for Harigian, who as a trainer helped sculpt some of Hollywood's finest bodies. "It has to be a room you want to be in," said Harigian.

Although rehabilitation for a college knee injury prompted him to change his major from architecture to exercise physiology, Harigian's fascination with designing the total workout environ-

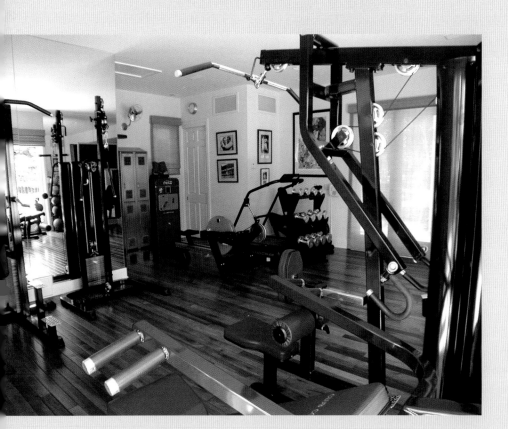

LEFT: Workout basics in this 1,000-square-foot Los Angeles gym include multi-station strength training equipment, a pulley cable station, a leg press, a rower, a treadmill, and cardio equipment. Every piece of equipment has been custom-sized for the client, whose home also includes a tennis/basketball court and pools. ABOVE RIGHT and FAR RIGHT: In this Grosse Point, Michigan, gym, installed over a four-car garage, a boxing bag covered in suede pivots alongside stainless steel laser-cut weight stacks. The client's name has been etched into each custom weight. The lockers in this gym were painted to match the vintage Pepsi cooler, while an antique rower serves as one-of-a-kind art when mounted on a blue background.

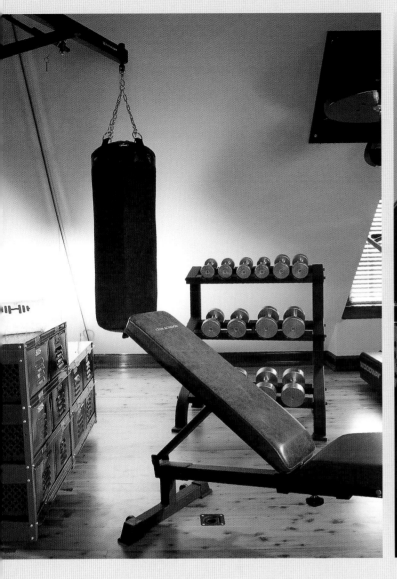

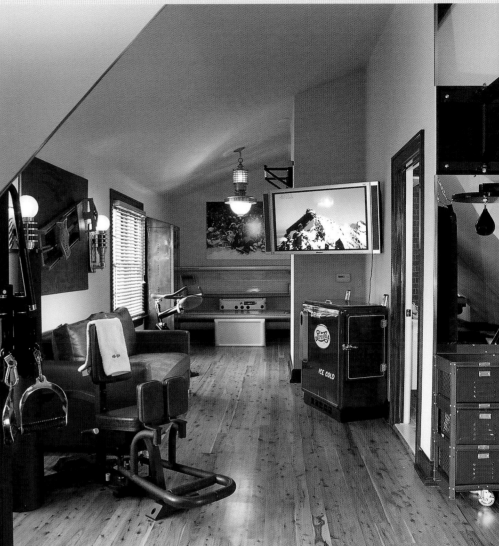

ment began while he was training celebrities in their homes. It heightened when his architect and designer clients would call him in for consultations on gym equipment.

While consulting on a gym for Tom Selleck's house, he noticed that the whole house was decorated in a Western ranch style but not the gym. So, he went to a saddle maker and requested custom pads for the gym equipment. He put in a rough, distressed floor. The interior designer loved it—and the rest was history.

In Harigian's gym designs, nothing is off the shelf, not even a pulley. Every bend, mold and custom part is made to exacting specifications. Although generic-sized equipment works for most people, custom equipment is extra important for, let's say, an NBA player. For Shaquille O'Neal, Harigian custom-built equip-

ment to scale, so the knees and elbows on O'Neal's seven-foot frame line up. "It's like the difference between buying a suit off the rack or having it tailor made for you," said Harigian.

After he sets up a gym, Harigian stays around to create an exercise video specifically of that person's workout routine, on their equipment and aimed at their specific goals. The video is timed so that he can cue his clients on to the next part of their exercise program.

If the price tag for Harigian's service (a starting fee of $75,000) exceeds some homeowners' budgets, the spirit with which he pursues his dreams and helps clients pursue their exercise goals may inspire a reshuffling of some home-design priorities.

"No other room in your house will do anything for your health," said Harigian.

And Then There Was Water

FOR THOSE WHO SECRETLY SUSPECT they are part mermen or mermaids—or for those whose physical condition or disability limits their ability to exercise—the kindest, most satisfying way to work out may be to embrace the buoyancy of water. Some very inspired interpretations of pool design can incite fantasies of growing fins, or at the very least encourage more laps across the pool.

A pool does not have to be merely the conventional shimmering square of water consigned to the backyard. A pool can be added indoors or outdoors—or be both, when divided into indoor and outdoor sections. Or a pool can be indoors and seem outdoors, like the shimmering wing designed by Bohlin Cywinski Jackson.

How about a pool on the roof, located so that exercise beckons every time you enter or leave the house? The architectural team of Messana O'Rorke created a pool on the second level of a home, which also serves as the entrance. Arriving home after a long run or a long day at work, a homeowner could hypothetically stop for a quick swim to cool off.

According to Brian Messana, this home was created for a client whose urban sensibilities conflict with her desire to live in the peace and quiet of the country. It was conceived as an island, a defensible oasis implanted gently in the midst of nature. Located north of New York City on an escarp-

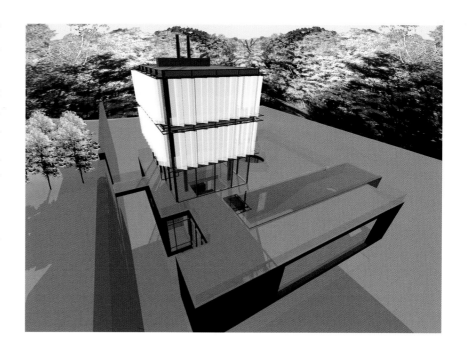

ment of a glacier-formed valley, this medieval-style building system might seem to require a moat but instead hovers over a meadow of wild flowers and grasses.

The island plain contains the home's living quarters—a free-flowing space where functions intermix--juxtaposed by a stand of mature maple trees that seem to pierce the structure. Breaks in the external envelope and a screened porch beneath the swimming pool provide long views out over the meadow to the woodlands beyond.

The roof is a garden that enjoys the upper boughs of the trees for shade and a lap pool, which is cantilevered out over the edge of the base. On this plateau, you enter the house

ABOVE: The second floor and yet entrance-level pool waits beside the home's front door as if beckoning the homeowner to toss aside that workday briefcase and jump right in. RIGHT: A style update on the moats that surrounded medieval castles, this swimming pool "moat" is designed to protect a homeowner from the effects of dietary excess by providing access to exercise. The architects describe the style of this home as a "defensible oasis."

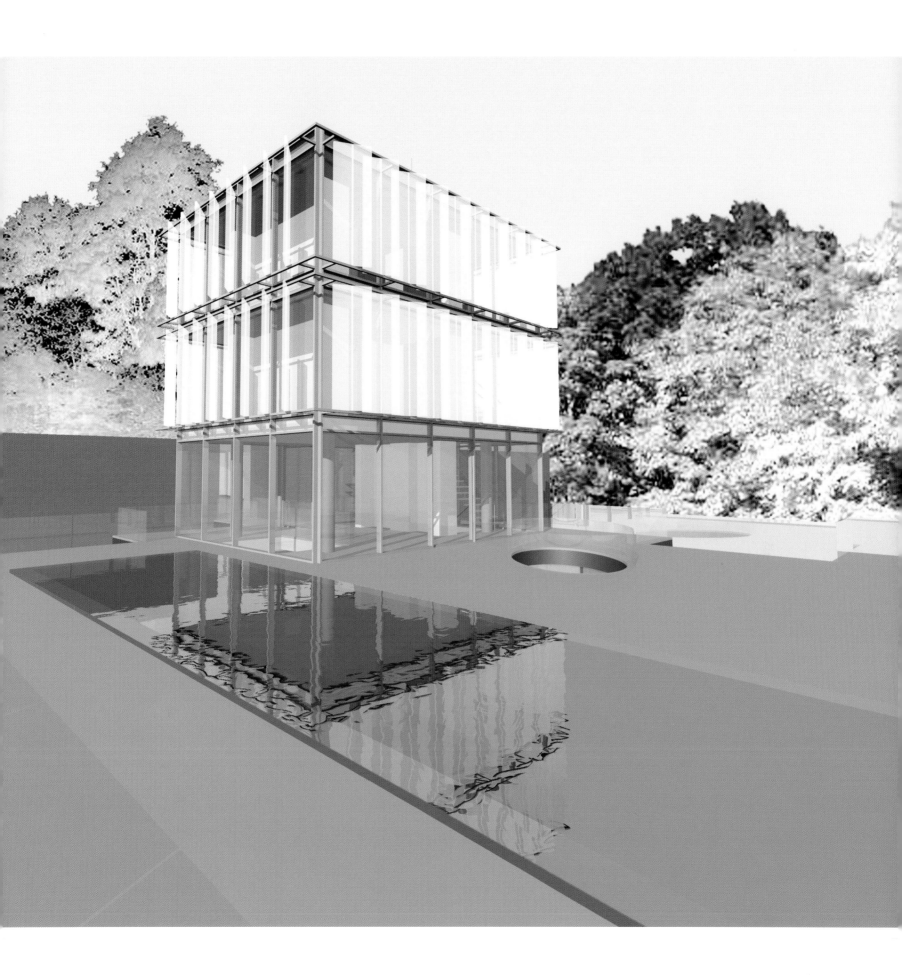

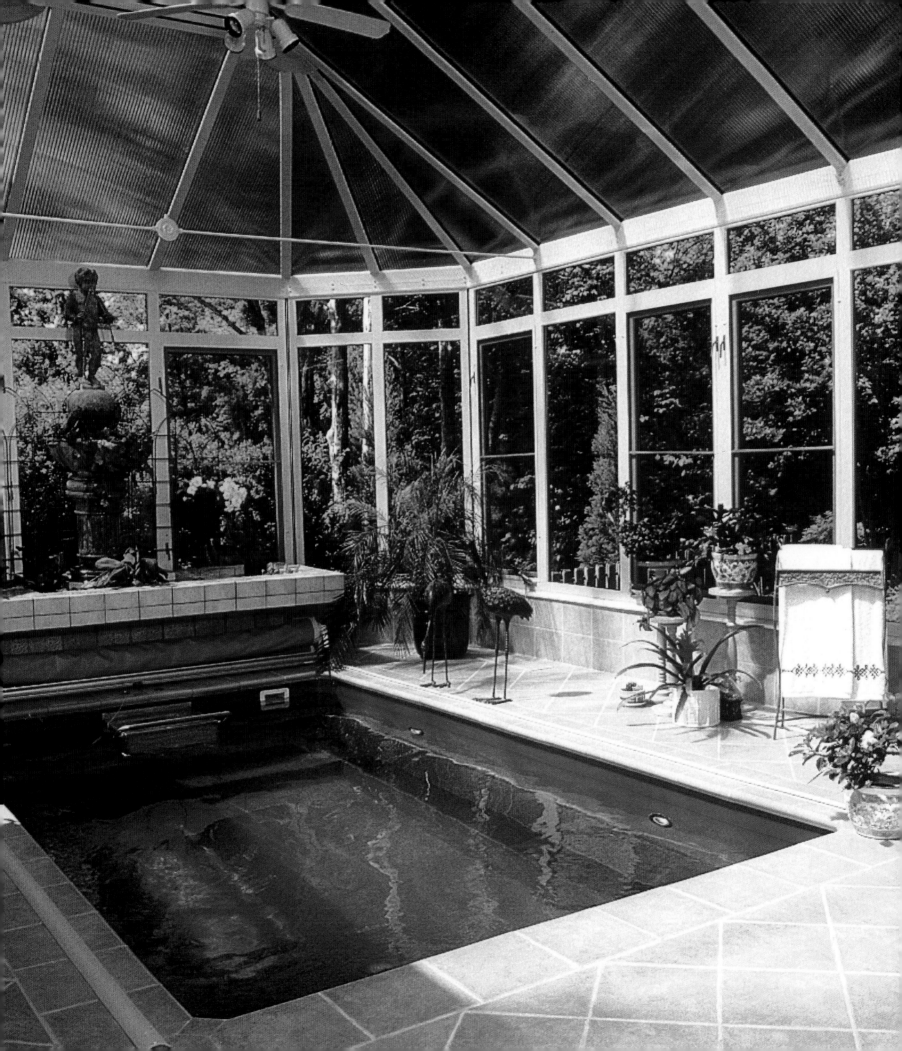

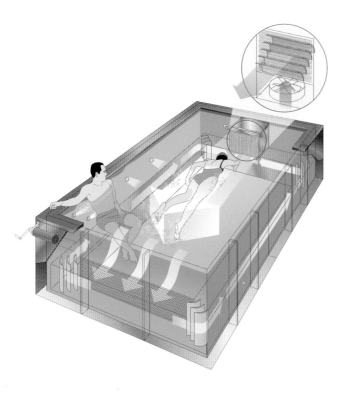

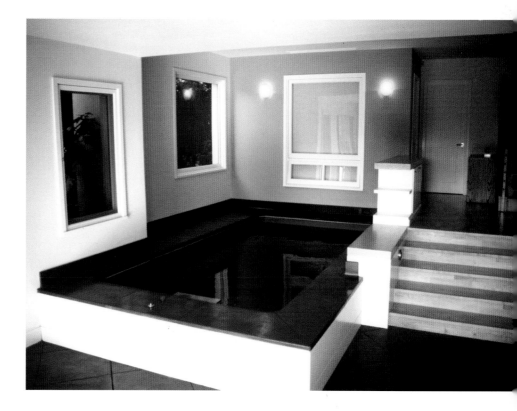

LEFT: A smaller space for a pool need not limit the benefits you get from swimming laps. With cross-current spa pools, you can swim in place and partake of the same exercise benefits you might get if you were crisscrossing a large pool. ABOVE: Swim-spa pools use a propeller system to create current. The effect of swimming in one of these pools is not unlike running on a treadmill. ABOVE RIGHT: Depending on your climate, budget, and confines, a small pool can be added in an enclosed backyard structure, in an addition, or even in a basement.

over a bridge from the top of the escarpment, between extended retaining walls.

Along the maple trees, a glass and steel medieval-inspired tower rises from the meadow through the solid form of the house and looks down over the garden. Rotating fiberglass sunscreens on the tower accommodate solar panels that enhance the heating and hot water needs of the house and provide additional privacy. The pool in itself is an island of serenity.

Creating Current

Although most spas are intended to soothe, a swim-spa combination may be especially useful if you don't have a lot of space for a pool. Adding current to a small pool can make it as efficient as a larger pool in which you swim laps.

To create calorie-burning, muscle-toning crosscurrent, swim-spa pools use a propeller system, jets, or a paddle wheel. Swimming against this current is not unlike running on a treadmill. With an average size of 14 to 15 feet long and 6 to 7 feet wide, a compact fiberglass, acrylic, or stainless steel pool with a vinyl liner can be incorporated into a previously underused space such as a basement or garage.

One way to improve on water exercise is to add more water—just for the sound effects. Few things are quite as soothing as the sound of running water. To add the voluptuous dimension of sound, a pool designer can incorporate a waterfall into a home pool or spa. Water can cascade over rocks, trickle from a suspended spout, or overflow gracefully, creating a fine, infinite silken sheet of liquid.

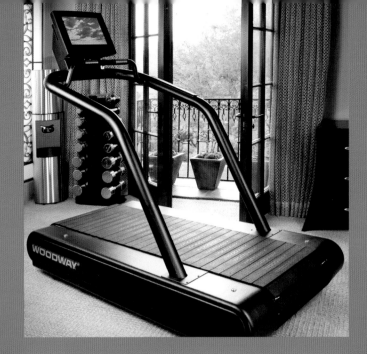

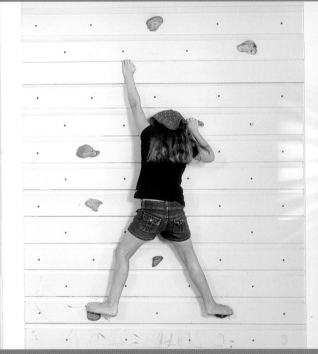

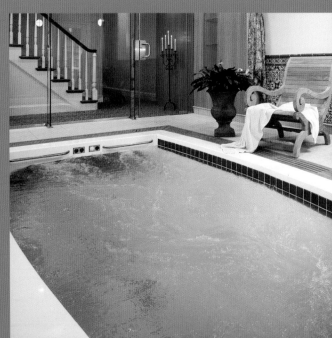

con

siderations

Gym Basics

WHEN PLANNING OR ADDING A HOME GYM, architects and designers now often consult gym-equipment professionals for advice on issues related to equipment, such as flooring and lighting. Most professionals and fitness experts agree that motivation is a key part of planning.

"The most important thing is to create a room that you want to be in. You have to do everything to motivate yourself, because people try to avoid exercise," says Richard Miller, president of Gym Source, which has set up gyms for three presidents and hyperbuff stars such as Madonna and Cher. For some that means eliminating distractions.

"The environment has to be conducive to getting away from distractions, away from the phone, the kids, away from the fridge," said fitness expert John Hanc, co-author of *The FORCE Program: The Proven Way to Fight Cancer Through Physical Activity and Exercise* and the author of several books on running. "It's the old story of the treadmill that ends up being a coat rack. Part of the reason that happens is because people don't create the proper environment."

To be inviting, ideally a workout room should have a high ceilings and lots of light and windows. Mirrors are a favored feature because they help create a feeling of space that's conducive to exercise. Mirrors also serve as a teaching tool if you work with a trainer.

According to Miller, color is an important consideration, since colors can stimulate adrenaline and increase motivation for certain types of energetic exercise. For example, red is highly motivational. Green is not, although it might be suited to a room in which yoga is practiced. The type of lighting chosen for a gym should not add too much heat or be too glaring.

One of the most important structural features in a home gym is ventilation. With a conventional air conditioner, the return on ventilation should be four times the normal amount. In terms of layout, placing the gym next to a pool can create problem moisture that can ultimately corrode gym equipment. This layout may necessitate additional moisture-removal considerations.

Gym floors should be pliant. Floors that bear the weight of exercise require more give. Just as walking on a treadmill is preferable to walking on concrete, since the cushioning reduces fatigue and reverberation, the same logic applies to selecting a floor material for your gym.

Tiles, concrete, and even industrial carpet over concrete may not offer enough resilience, says Miller. Residential carpets are too soft and do not offer stability, since exercise machines can sink into them. For an added degree of flexibility, wooden gym floors are often created using "sleepers," pieces of studs that raise the wooden floor from the concrete.

"While wood floors offer the best aesthetic appeal, they are not always best," said Miller. "You might be able to go with wood floors on a second-floor gym, but you need a rubber gym floor, especially over cement. However, not all rubber flooring is alike. Some cannot stand up to the weight of the machines."

Ideally, rubber flooring should be at least three-quarters of an inch thick. Besides being low maintenance, rubber flooring can also help even out a floor that is not quite smooth. If you do decide to install a carpet, say, in an upstairs home gym, select one made of natural fibers, since synthetic carpets in a workout environment may promote the growth of bacteria.

Although a workout room should be free from stimuli that can keep you from exercising, some types of distractions may be welcome. Surprisingly, says Miller, most gym layouts start with a piece of equipment that many fault as a reason more people are going to the gym—the TV.

"Most people like to work out with external stimuli, such as music for motivation," said Hanc. When working on cardio equipment, many exercisers like to watch TV, so in gym planning, the first fixed point may be the location of the set.

When setting up a home gym, professionals start by asking clients what kind of exercise they like and what equipment they use in a gym, how often they exercise, and how fitness works best in their lifestyle.

To combat the high-stress, sedentary lifestyles so many people are prey to, three types of exercise are optimum—cardiovascular or cardio, strength training, and flexibility training. For cardio the trendiest piece of equipment is the elliptical, which incorporates the sideways, up-and-down movements of several types of machines. The second most popular piece of equipment is the treadmill. For strength training, there are weights that can be adjusted to various weights and benches for use with dumbbells. For flexibility, many people practice yoga or Pilates, but a medicine or Swiss ball, a foam mat for the floor, and stretching ropes can form the basics of a stretching program.

According to Hanc, a marathon runner, if you had to get one piece of fitness equipment to start with, the best bet might be the treadmill. "Making this piece of home equipment affordable was a major step in home fitness," said Hanc, "because it allows people to engage in the most basic and available fitness activity—which is walking—and that's, funny as it sounds, a big step forward."

Exercise equipment can be customized with additional features or be built from scratch to fit into a specific space. One Gym Source client had a piece of equipment designed to fold into the wall under a panel papered the same way as the rest of the room.

Before a gym is outfitted, the experts make a floor plan using specialized computer software to block out various types of equipment, maximize views and, if necessary, provide adequate space for more than one person to use the equipment at the same time.

How much space do you really need? It depends on your interests and budget. Even small spaces can incorporate some element of fitness, whether it's a medicine ball, a yoga mat, or a folding treadmill. For maximum effect, professionals recommend an exercise space no smaller than 200 square feet. Even for two pieces of cardio equipment, a weight bench, and dumbbells, you need at least 120 square feet of space and a ceiling that's 7 or 8 feet high. The American Council on Exercise offers the following guidelines for installing equipment:

TREADMILLS	30 square feet
SINGLE-STATION GYM	35 square feet
FREE WEIGHTS	20 to 50 square feet
BIKES	10 square feet
ROWING MACHINES	20 square feet
STAIR CLIMBERS	10 to 20 square feet
SKI MACHINES	25 square feet
MULTI-STATION GYM	50 to 200 square feet

When planning a gym, be sure to designate enough floor space for adding equipment in the future. On the other hand, it may be prudent to start with only one or two pieces of equipment and see if you are really going to use them.

The best way to avoid gym equipment becoming impromptu coat hangers, says Miller, is not to buy substandard equipment. As with anything else, you get what you pay for. Buying equipment from a reputable company that maintains it may insure equipment longevity.

The Federal Trade Commission (FTC) suggests evaluating claims carefully before buying any exercise equipment. No matter what an advertisement says, the only way exercise equipment can be effective is for you to use it.

"No machine can exercise for you," said Hanc. "A simple exercise mat is more effective than a $10,000 home set up if a person uses the exercise mat as opposed to not using equipment."

When buying equipment, read the fine print. Get the details on warranties, guarantees, and return policies. Gym equipment should have a warranty of at least six months. Be sure service is included in your warranty, since gym equipment requires more service than any other purchase, except perhaps cars.

If you are considering buying a piece of exercise equipment secondhand, check www.cpsc.gov to see if the equipment has been recalled.

Children and Exercise Equipment

Scaled-down versions of exercise equipment for children now approach the popularity of adult fitness equipment. It's a misguided idea to hold children up to adult workout standards or to let children work out—even on child-size equipment—alone, says Hanc. Parents should always supervise any strength-training exercises such as weight lifting and bench presses. Children can injure themselves by lifting weights that are too heavy or by dropping heavy equipment on themselves.

It is a smart idea to keep small children away from adult exercise equipment in which they could get their fingers caught. The United States Consumer Product Safety Commission (CPSC) estimates that each year about 8,700 children under five years of age are injured by getting their fingers caught in adult exercise equipment. Some of the biggest offenders include stationary bicycles, treadmills, and stair climbers. To prevent such injuries, never use an exercise bike without a chain guard. Store bikes away when not in use.

Before Taking The Plunge

Deciding you want a pool may be the easy part. Then you have to decide whether to have an indoor or outdoor pool and what type of pool. Climate and use are the most important considerations, with outdoor pools being most popular where they can be used most of the year. To help determine length and depth, decide how you will use your pool. Will you swim laps? Perform aqua aerobics?

If you decide on an in-ground outdoor pool, climate and geographical conditions may further determine which type you choose: concrete, vinyl lined, or fiberglass. Fiberglass pools, generally installed in one piece, may be more expensive than concrete, but tend to last longer and need less maintenance. Fiberglass also has a shock-absorbent quality that suits earthquake-prone areas, such as California.

Concrete pools are the most common. Although they cost less and are easier to customize, they take longer to install. Concrete pools require excavation, steel installation, plumbing, and finishing applications, such as tile, paint, or decorative pebbles.

Adding a vinyl liner, in-ground pool requires digging a hole, fastening panel walls together, and supporting the bottom with a concrete footing. The vinyl liner is spread over the inside of the pool and connected to the panels. Installation takes only a few weeks, but depending on the climate, liners may need to be replaced periodically.

Indoor pools are usually made from concrete and are part of the design and structure of the building in which they are located. Although the pool may require heating, placing it in direct sunshine can help cut heating costs. Installing a solar heating system that means solar energy can be used to warm the pool.

Outdoor pools are best integrated into the landscape, either placed where they fit into the footprint of the home's surrounding grounds and gardens or where they take advantage of the natural terrain. Living near an expansive view or, best yet, a body of water offers the opportunity of placing the pool so it seems to visually blend into the horizon.

Working with a Contractor

When you are planning to add a pool, it's wise to find out what building permits are needed. Zoning requirements may dictate any pool specifics, such as how high a pool's surrounding fence can be or how far from the property line a pool can be built. Once such paperwork is dealt with, the next step is making a budget.

When calculating the price, don't forget to factor in any potential extras, such as fencing and landscaping. Are electrical work, plumbing and masonry factored into the installation price? If you plan on doing any part of the project yourself, you may want to get an estimate on materials. It's also more cost efficient to install an outdoor pool before any landscaping is done, so it can be coordinated with any garden drip-irrigation systems.

It's essential to consider safety. Will the pool be fenced off to protect small, curious children or pets? If you can see the fence from inside the home, what's the visual impact? Also, with an outdoor pool, be sure to plan adequate deck area for lounging, pool furniture, and meals al fresco. When hiring a pool installer, ask for more than one reference, and always ask about a warranty.

Moisture Control

If you are building an indoor pool, it's a good idea to ask how the installer or architect will deal with moisture control.

"If you don't have the right kind of moisture-control system on an indoor pool, you can have major problems," said John Martin of John Martin Associates Architects in Torrington,

Connecticut. "Moisture can cause wood to rot." Be sure to include the price of moisture-control systems in your budget, since they can often cost as much as the pool itself. Some systems, however, can put the heat generated by the motor to good use by warming the pool.

Spa Safety

Although the purpose of a spa is to relax and revitalize you, personal spas can be hazardous if they are not used properly. About 700 deaths are reported each year from spa drownings. When drains get blocked, the obstruction can cause the spa's pump to work harder, resulting in greater suction, which in turn causes the entanglements that can lead to drowning. By choosing a spa with two suction openings or drains for each pump, you can reduce the risk, because this arrangement lessens the amount of suction for each pump.

For safety's sake, the Underwriter's Laboratories (UL) suggest that spa owners:

- Never operate a spa if suction fittings are broken or missing
- Keep water temperature at 104 degrees Fahrenheit or below
- Never use the spa while under the influence of drugs or alcohol
- Know where the cut-off switch for the pump is in case of an emergency
- Attach a locked spa cover after each use
- Never soak in a spa alone
- Supervise children at all times
- To prevent electrocution, never place any electric appliance within five feet of the spa
- Consult your doctor before using a spa if you are pregnant

Keeping Your Pool Clean

Although nothing kills all of the germs that grow in pools and spas, chlorine can sanitize 99 percent of the germs in a matter of seconds. However, several side effects of chlorine are not very appealing, including its smell, the way it can irritate sensitive skin or eyes, and the way it prematurely fades bathing suits. A number of alternative sanitizers are currently available. An increasingly popular alternative is biguanide (PHMB), first developed as a presurgery antimicrobial scrub. An effective germ killer, PHMB is gentler on the skin and eyes than chlorine. Its primary drawback is that it can cost up to 20 percent more than chlorine.

Healthy Building Materials

Staying healthy means more than just strengthening and nourishing your body. It also involves protecting your body from potentially hazardous pollutants. Ideally, the high fit home does not endanger the health of its occupants through the use of inherently hazardous building materials. A key ingredient in building healthy homes is the use of healthy building materials, including those made without PVC (polyvinyl chloride) or formaldehyde, or with no or low VOCs (volatile organic compounds). Healthy materials are safely reusable, recyclable, or biodegradable.

There's also a growing concern about protecting the world's old-growth forests. The average home contains more than 10,000 board feet of framing lumber. Homeowners are becoming more aware that razing forests to build human homes may endanger the natural habitat of other living things. To promote the health of the planet—to preserve biodiversity and help minimize the threat of global warming—many home builders seek alternatives to using wood from old-growth forests. Recommended alternatives include certified sustainable wood, composition or engineered wood products, salvaged or reclaimed wood, and recycled materials.

The High Fit Home

For a high fit home to be your home, it must reflect what's important to you. Although a home cannot force anyone to be healthy or stay fit, it can make a strong statement about priorities and promote fitness values. As people strive for a personal physical ideal, they can find positive reinforcement and encouragement in their immediate environment.

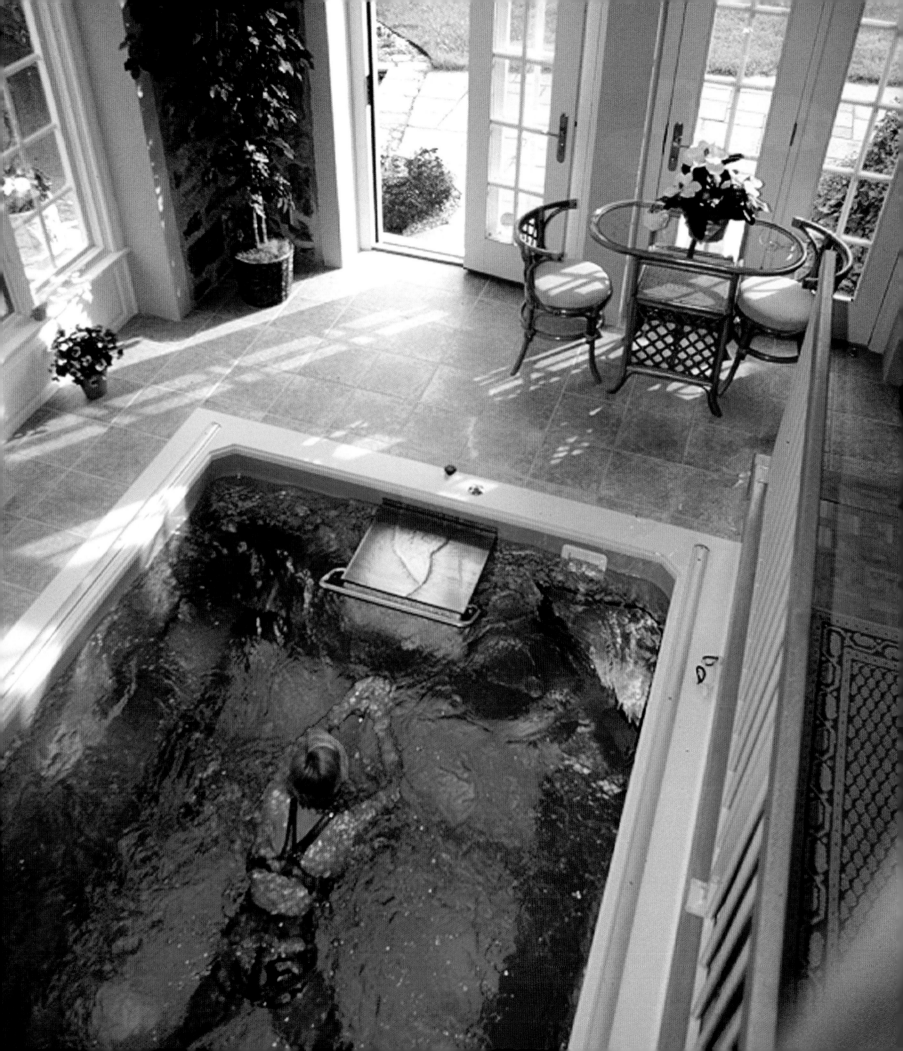

Abramson Teiger Architects
8924 Lindblade Street
Culver City, California 90232
310-838-8998 telephone
310-838-8332 fax
trevor@abramsonteiger.com
douglas@abramsonteiger.com
www.abramsonteiger.com

Ahmann Architects
4408 Beechwood Road
University Park, Maryland 02782
301-864-1334 telephone
AhmannArch@aol.com

Alison Brooks Architects Ltd.
Unit 610 Highgate Studios
53-79 Highgate Road
London NW5 1TL
England
44-020-7267-9777 telephone
44-020-7267-9772 fax
www.alisonbrooksarchitects.com

Anderson Anderson Architecture
83 Columbia Street, Suite 300
Seattle, Washington 98104
206-332-9500 telephone
415-520-9522 fax

ALSO:
90 Tehama Street
San Francisco, California 94105
415-243-9500 telephone
415-520-9522 fax
info@andersonanderson.com
www.andersonanderson.com

Andrew Pilkington Architects
382–386 Edgware Road
London W2 1EB
England
44-020-7402-4013 telephone
info@andrewpilkington.com
www.andrewpilkington.com

Architectenbureau Jaco D. De Visser
Oudegracht 316
3511PK Utrecht
The Netherlands
31-030-231-9892 telephone
31-030-232-1657 fax
jaco@devisserbv.nl
www.devisserbv.nl

archi-tectonics
200 Varick Sreet, Suite 507B
New York, New York 10014
212-226-0303 telephone
212-219-3106 fax
info@archi-tectonics.com
www.archi-tectonics.com

Bohlin Cywinski Jackson
8 West Market Street, Suite 1200
Wilkes-Barre, Pennsylvania 18701
570-825-8756 telephone
570-825-3744 fax
www.bcj.com

ALSO:
307 Fourth Avenue , Suite 1300
Pittsburgh, Pennsylvania 15222
412-765-3890 telephone
412-765-2209 fax

ALSO:
123 South Broad Street , Suite 1370
Philadelphia, Pennsylvania 19109
215-790-5900 telephone
215-790-5901 fax

ALSO:
1932 First Avenue, Suite 916
Seattle, Washington 98101
206-256-0862 telephone
206-256-0864 fax

ALSO:
733 Allston Way
Berkeley, California 94710
510-841-5564 telephone
510-841-5090 fax
www.bcj.com

Bryden Wood Associates
15 Bowling Green Lane
London EC1R 0BD
England
44-020-7253-4772 telephone
44-020-7253-4773 fax
bwa@brydenwood.co.uk
www.brydenwood.co.uk

Camille Urban Jobe Architecture
1000 North Rainbow Ranch Road
Wimberly, Texas 78676
www.urbanjobe.com
512-585-3466 telephone
cjobe@urbanjobe.com

Cheryl Gardner, I.D.
569 North Rossmore Avenue, Suite 607
Los Angeles, California 90004
323-856-0812 telephone
323-856-4241 fax

ALSO:
701 Fourth Avenue South
Minneapolis, Minnesota 55414
612-333-2602 telephone
www.cherylgardner.com
cheryl@cherylgardner.com

Eric Owen Moss
8557 Higuera Street
Culver City, California 90232
310-839-1199 telephone
310-839-7922 fax
mail@ericowenmoss.com
www.ericowenmoss.com

Endless Pools, Inc.
200 East Dutton Mill Road
Aston, Pennsylvania 19014
800-732-8660
610-497-8676 telephone
610-497-9328 fax
swim@endlesspools.com
www.endlesspools.com

Ethelind Coblin Architect, P.C.
505 Eighth Avenue, Suite 2202
New York, New York 10018
212-967-2490 telephone
212-967-2197 fax
ecoblin@ecapcaia.com
www.newyork-architects.com/ecoblin

Everlast Climbing Industries
3140 Neil Armstrong Boulevard, Suite 304
Eagan, Minnesota 55121
800-476-7366
www.traversewall.com

Graftworks Architecture + Design
1123 Broadway, Suite 715
New York, New York 10010
212-366-9675 telephone
212-366-9075 fax
www.graftworks.net
info@graftworks.net

Gray Organschi Architecture
78 Olive Street
New Haven, Connecticut 06511
203-777-7794 telephone
203-782-0940 fax
kyle@grayorganschi.com
www.grayorganschi.com

Grimshaw Architects
1 Conway Street
Fitzroy Square
London W1T6LR
England
44-020-7291-4141 telephone
44-020-7291-4194 fax
www.grimshaw-architects.com

Grimshaw (USA)
100 Reade Street
New York, New York 10013
212-791-2581 telephone
212-791-2173 fax

Gym Source
800-GYM-SOURCE
info@gymsource.com
www.gymsource.com

HammerSmith, Inc.
807 Church Street
Decatur, Georgia 30030
404-377-1021 telephone
404-377-9827 fax
renovate@hammersmith.net
www.hammersmith.net

Harigian Fitness
11718 Barrington Court, Suite 138
Los Angeles, California 90049
310-366-3297 telephone
www.harigianfitness.com

Joel Sanders, Architect
515 Canal Street
New York, New York 10013
212-431-8751 telephone
212-225-9486 fax
info@joelsandersarchitect.com
www.joelsandersarchitect.com

John Martin Associates Architects
760 East Main Street
Torrington, Connecticut 06790
860-496-1233 telephone
860-496-7343 fax
martinarchitects@snet.net

Konyk
61 Pearl Street, Suite 509
Brooklyn, New York 11201
718-852-5381 telephone
718-852-1890 fax
konyl@konyk.net
www.konyk.net

Lee Wimpenny Design Associates
31 Bleecker Street
New York, New York 10012
212-505-8408 telephone
212-529-8833 fax
www.leewimpenny.com

Louise Braverman, Architect
16 East 79th Street, Suite 43
New York, New York 10021
212-879-6155 telephone
212-879-3492 fax

Messana O'Rorke Architects
118 West 22nd Street
Ninth Floor
New York, New York 10011
212-807-1960 telephone
212-807-1966 fax
brian@messanaororke.com
www.messanaororke.com

MKarchitecture
Berkeley, California
415-999-4122 telephone
michelle@mkarchitecture
www.mkarchitecture.com

Murdock Young Architects
526 West 26th Street, Suite 616
New York, New York 10011
212-924-9775 telephone
212-924-9865 fax
www.murdockyoung.com

Naomi Leff and Associates, Inc.
12 West 27th Street
New York, New York 10001
212-686-6300 telephone
212-213-9208 fax
www.naomileff.com

Resolution: 4 Architecture
150 West 28th Street, Suite 1902
New York, New York 10001
212-675-9266 telephone
info@RE4A.com
www.re4a.com

SwimEx
373 Market Street
Warren, Rhode Island 02885
800-877-7946 telephone
401-245-3160 fax
www.swimex.com